Emmanuel Obeng-Gyasi
Joav Merrick
Editors

Public Health

Understanding the Impact of Environmental Pollutants

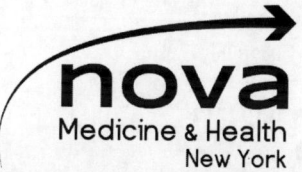

Copyright © 2025 by Nova Science Publishers, Inc.
DOI: https://doi.org/10.52305/YJZT4514

All rights reserved. No part of this book may be reproduced, stored in a retrieval system or transmitted in any form or by any means: electronic, electrostatic, magnetic, tape, mechanical photocopying, recording or otherwise without the written permission of the Publisher.

We have partnered with Copyright Clearance Center to make it easy for you to obtain permissions to reuse content from this publication. Simply navigate to this publication's page on Nova's website and locate the "Get Permission" button below the title description. This button is linked directly to the title's permission page on copyright.com. Alternatively, you can visit copyright.com and search by title, ISBN, or ISSN.

For further questions about using the service on copyright.com, please contact:
Copyright Clearance Center
Phone: +1-(978) 750-8400   Fax: +1-(978) 750-4470   E-mail: info@copyright.com.

NOTICE TO THE READER

The Publisher has taken reasonable care in the preparation of this book, but makes no expressed or implied warranty of any kind and assumes no responsibility for any errors or omissions. No liability is assumed for incidental or consequential damages in connection with or arising out of information contained in this book. The Publisher shall not be liable for any special, consequential, or exemplary damages resulting, in whole or in part, from the readers' use of, or reliance upon, this material. Any parts of this book based on government reports are so indicated and copyright is claimed for those parts to the extent applicable to compilations of such works.

Independent verification should be sought for any data, advice or recommendations contained in this book. In addition, no responsibility is assumed by the Publisher for any injury and/or damage to persons or property arising from any methods, products, instructions, ideas or otherwise contained in this publication.

The Publisher assumes no responsibility for any statements of fact or opinion expressed in the published contents.

This publication is designed to provide accurate and authoritative information with regard to the subject matter covered herein. It is sold with the clear understanding that the Publisher is not engaged in rendering legal or any other professional services. If legal or any other expert assistance is required, the services of a competent person should be sought. FROM A DECLARATION OF PARTICIPANTS JOINTLY ADOPTED BY A COMMITTEE OF THE AMERICAN BAR ASSOCIATION AND A COMMITTEE OF PUBLISHERS.

Additional color graphics may be available in the e-book version of this book.

Library of Congress Cataloging-in-Publication Data

ISBN: 979-8-89530-579-9 (Softcover)
ISBN: 979-8-89530-636-9 (e-Book)

Published by Nova Science Publishers, Inc. † New York

Contents

Introduction 1

Chapter 1 Understanding the impact of environmental
pollutants on public health 3
Emmanuel Obeng-Gyasi and Joav Merrick

Section One: Environmetal health 7

Chapter 2 Empowering communities:
The role of wearable devices
in environmental justice 9
*Akua Marfo
and Emmanuel Obeng-Gyasi*

Chapter 3 Occupational determinants of health 55
*Aderonke Adetunji
and Emmanuel Obeng-Gyasi*

Chapter 4 How combined PFAS (per- and polyfluoroalkyl
substances) and metals may contribute
to chronic obstructive pulmonary disease 85
Aderonke Ayodele and Emmanuel Obeng-Gyasi

Chapter 5 A review on the potential lead pollution
in domestic water use in the State
of Mississippi 99
*William Dodoo Sackey
and Emmanuel Obeng-Gyasi*

Chapter 6 Association of mercury exposure with allostatic
load and cardiovascular disease risk 113
Hayley Howard and Emmanuel Obeng-Gyasi

Chapter 7	Association of total arsenic exposure with allostatic load and cardiovascular disease risk .... 131 Elon Barbee and Emmanuel Obeng-Gyasi	

Section Two: Acknowledgments 149

Chapter 8	About the Authors 151
Chapter 9	About the Department of Built Environment, North Carolina A&T State University, Greensboro and Environmental Health and Disease Laboratory, North Carolina A&T State University, Greensboro, North Carolina, United States of America 153
Chapter 10	About the National Institute of Child Health and Human Development in Israel 155

Section Three: Index 159

Index 161

Introduction

Chapter 1

Understanding the impact of environmental pollutants on public health

Emmanuel Obeng-Gyasi[1,2,*], PhD, MPH and Joav Merrick[3-6], MD, MMedSci, DMSc

[1]Department of Built Environment and [2]Environmental Health and Disease Laboratory, North Carolina A&T State University, Greensboro, North Carolina, United States of America
[3]National Institute of Child Health and Human Development, Jerusalem, Israel
[4]Department of Pediatrics, Mt Scopus Campus, Hadassah Medical Center and Faculty of Medicine, Hebrew University of Jerusalem, Jerusalem, Israel
[5]Kentucky Children's Hospital, University of Kentucky, Lexington, Kentucky, United States of America
[6]Center for Healthy Development, School of Public Health, Georgia State University, Atlanta, United States of America

Abstract

Research on environmental pollutants underscores a significant public health issue across various sectors and populations. The research provides crucial insights into how occupational exposures and widespread environmental contaminants play a crucial role in shaping health outcomes, with a particular focus on the risks associated with arsenic and mercury, the health hazards in the various industries and the transformative power of technology to mitigate these risks.

---

[*] *Correspondence:* Emmanuel Obeng-Gyasi, PhD, MPH, Department of Built Environment, North Carolina A&T State University, Greensboro and Environmental Health and Disease Laboratory, North Carolina A&T State University, Greensboro, North Carolina 27411, United States of America. Email: eobenggyasi@ncat.edu

In: Public Health: Understanding the Impact of Environmental Pollutants
Editors: Emmanuel Obeng-Gyasi and Joav Merrick
ISBN: 979-8-89530-579-9
© 2025 Nova Science Publishers, Inc.

Introduction

The growing body of research on environmental pollutants underscores a significant public health crisis that spans across various sectors and populations. This body of work provides crucial insights into how occupational exposures and widespread environmental contaminants play a crucial role in shaping health outcomes, with a particular focus on the risks associated with arsenic and mercury, the health hazards in the various industries, and the transformative power of technology to mitigate these risks.

The cardiovascular risks of arsenic and mercury exposure

The assessment of the cardiovascular risks associated with exposure to arsenic and mercury are influenced by the mediums through which these pollutants are measured, such as blood and urine. This is crucial because the half-life of these pollutants differs significantly in these mediums, which may affect the detection and interpretation of results. For instance, mercury is known to accumulate in the human body and can be reliably measured in blood, reflecting long-term exposure. In contrast, arsenic's presence in urine might only indicate recent exposure due to its shorter half-life in this medium.

These variations in measurement can lead to complexities in understanding how each pollutant contributes to cardiovascular diseases. Both arsenic and mercury are associated with cardiovascular risks through mechanisms like oxidative stress and inflammation, but the impact of the testing medium highlights the need for precise and context-specific research methods. This underscores the importance of careful consideration in choosing the appropriate biomarkers for environmental health studies, aiming to ensure accurate assessments of exposure and risk.

Understanding health outcomes in occupational environments

Occupational health risks extend far beyond any single industry, affecting various sectors with profound implications for worker health and safety. These risks are often exacerbated in environments where workers face significant exposures to hazardous substances. The determinants of health in these occupational settings include physical factors such as exposure to toxic chemicals and dyes, ergonomic challenges from repetitive tasks, and psychosocial stresses including long working hours and job insecurity.

For instance, workers in various industries often come into contact with a range of chemicals that can cause respiratory issues, skin irritation, and long-term conditions such as cancer and cardiovascular diseases. Moreover, the psychosocial stressors associated with occupational settings, such as low job control, high job demands, and lack of support, can lead to both physical and mental health problems, including cardiovascular diseases, depression, and anxiety. These conditions highlight the critical need for comprehensive workplace health policies that encompass health promotion, disease prevention, and worker empowerment initiatives to address these broad determinants of health.

Improving occupational health also involves regulatory oversight to ensure safe working conditions, regular health screenings to monitor the effects of occupational exposures, and ongoing education on safe practices. Additionally, enhancing the physical and mental well-being of workers by addressing these occupational determinants of health can significantly contribute to overall public health and productivity.

Wearable devices: Advancing health equity in environmental monitoring

Advancements in technology are revolutionizing how we address environmental justice, particularly through the use of wearable devices. These devices provide a novel means to monitor individual exposures to environmental pollutants and offer unprecedented opportunities to close the environmental justice gap. Wearable technology enables real-time data collection on environmental exposures, such as air quality and noise levels, directly affecting individuals in their daily lives.

In underserved communities, which often bear the brunt of environmental injustices due to proximity to industrial sites and high pollution areas, wearable devices can play a critical role. They provide tangible evidence that can support community claims about disproportionate exposure to pollutants. This data becomes a powerful tool in advocating for policy changes and remedial actions to address these disparities.

Moreover, wearable devices empower individuals by making them active participants in monitoring and managing their health relative to environmental factors. For example, residents in areas with poor air quality can use wearable air quality monitors to avoid outdoor activities during times of high pollution. This capability not only enhances individual health outcomes but also fosters a greater awareness of the link between the environment and health among community members.

Furthermore, the data collected through these devices can be used to create more targeted public health interventions. By analyzing trends over time, health officials can identify which interventions are most effective and where they are needed the most, thus optimizing resource allocation and intervention strategies.

Section One: Environmetal health

Chapter 2

Empowering communities: The role of wearable devices in environmental justice

**Akua Marfo, BA
and Emmanuel Obeng-Gyasi*, PhD, MPH**
Department of Built Environment and Environmental Health and Disease Laboratory, North Carolina A&T State University, Greensboro, North Carolina, United States of America

Abstract

This chapter delves into the emerging role of wearable devices in the realm of environmental justice and public health monitoring, offering a novel perspective on how technology can empower communities, especially those facing disproportionate environmental challenges. It provides an in-depth analysis of various wearable sensor technologies, including air quality monitors, UV exposure sensors, and water quality sensors, highlighting their significance in real-time environmental and health data collection. The research underscores the importance of these devices in enabling marginalized communities to actively participate in monitoring and responding to environmental health hazards. By facilitating access to personalized and location-specific environmental data, wearable technologies not only raise individual awareness but also contribute to community-level advocacy and action. Furthermore, the

---

* *Correspondence:* Associate professor Emmanuel Obeng-Gyasi, PhD, MPH, Department of Built Environment and Environmental Health and Disease Laboratory, North Carolina A&T State University, Greensboro, North C 27411, United States of America. Email: eobenggyasi@ncat.edu

In: Public Health: Understanding the Impact of Environmental Pollutants
Editors: Emmanuel Obeng-Gyasi and Joav Merrick
ISBN: 979-8-89530-579-9
© 2025 Nova Science Publishers, Inc.

paper explores the potential advancements in wearable technologies through the integration of AI and machine learning, enhancing their effectiveness in data analysis and interpretation. However, it also critically examines the challenges associated with data privacy, security, and accessibility, emphasizing the need for inclusive and equitable technology deployment. This study is significant for its contribution to understanding the intersection of technology, environmental health, and social justice. It argues that wearable devices can be transformative tools in achieving environmental justice, providing communities with the means to gather evidence, advocate for change, and protect public health. The findings of this paper are pertinent for policymakers, public health officials, and environmental justice advocates seeking to leverage technology for societal benefit.

Introduction

Environmental justice (EJ) is defined by the US Environmental Protection Agency (USEPA) as the equitable treatment and meaningful involvement of all individuals, irrespective of "race, color, national origin, or income, in the development, implementation, and enforcement of environmental laws, regulations, and policies" (1).

EJ studies scholar Robert Bullard defines environmental justice as a principle of "equal protection and equal enforcement of our environmental, health, housing, land use, transportation, energy, and civil rights laws and regulation" (2).

EJ means every individual should be protected, and no group should be disadvantaged or suffer the impact of environmental issues. Individuals, whether majority, minority, rich or poor should have the opportunity to live in a clean and unpolluted environment. EJ is not only about protecting the population from environmental conditions but also about creating a clean and safe environment for individuals to thrive and enjoy a good life.

The EJ movement is often recognized as having its roots in the 1982 Warren County protest in North Carolina. This significant event marked a pivotal moment in civil rights and environmental activism, as it brought together a diverse coalition of residents, civil rights activists, and political leaders. They united in response to the proposed construction of a landfill site for the disposal of soil contaminated with polychlorinated biphenyls (PCBs), a group of highly toxic chemicals. This proposal came after the discovery that over 32,000 cubic yards of PCB-contaminated soil had been illegally dumped along roadways in fourteen North Carolina counties in 1978. The protest in Warren County, a community significantly impacted by these actions, stands as a landmark event in the ongoing struggle for environmental justice and equity, highlighting the intersection of racial, social, and environmental issues (3).

Even though the protest in Warren County did not ultimately prevent the disposal of PCBs in the area, it nevertheless succeeded in raising the issue of environmental justice to national and international prominence (4). This movement was crucial in spotlighting environmental injustices, particularly how they disproportionately affect marginalized communities in the United States. Following the protest, there was a heightened governmental and scholarly focus on understanding and addressing environmental disparities. This increased attention led to extensive research into the patterns, impacts, and potential solutions for environmental inequities, especially in historically underserved areas.

Research findings over the years have consistently highlighted a troubling trend: communities with predominantly African American populations and those of lower socio-economic status were more likely to be selected for the disposal of hazardous waste. This practice not only posed severe environmental risks but also had significant health implications for the residents of these areas. The Warren County protest thus stands as a landmark event in the ongoing efforts to achieve environmental justice and equality, shedding light on the intersection of environmental issues with racial and socio-economic factors (5). This recognition further emphasized the need for comprehensive action to rectify these injustices.

Numerous essential research studies have outlined that individuals from marginalized communities, including people of color, those with lower socioeconomic status, indigenous and immigrant populations, are disproportionately impacted by environmentally harmful infrastructures. These infrastructures include landfills, mines, incinerators, polluting factories, and disruptive transportation systems. Additionally, these communities bear a higher burden of negative consequences stemming from ecologically harmful practices, such as climate change/disruption and pesticide exposure (6).

Inhabitants of marginalized communities face the dire consequences of environmental injustice, primarily due to their limited access to costly, advanced tools for assessing environmental pollutants. Furthermore, their reliance on governmental authorities to gauge pollution levels often results in agonizingly slow responses (7). State-provided environmental monitoring methods, including air and water quality assessments, soil sampling, and noise pollution evaluations, can be resource-intensive and often inefficient in timely service delivery to impacted communities. It is increasingly critical for residents in marginalized areas to adopt cost-effective, personal monitoring tools to assess environmental pollution levels. This approach not only facilitates a more direct understanding of pollution's impact but also empowers these communities to advocate effectively against detrimental environmental decisions.

Wearable environmental monitoring devices can offer a practical solution, particularly for residents in underserved communities. These devices are capable of tracking a range of environmental parameters, such as air quality, temperature, and humidity, directly in the wearer's immediate surroundings. By employing these tools, individuals can obtain real-time data on the extent of environmental pollution, providing a basis for informed community action.

This strategy represents a shift from relying solely on traditional, often costly, state-managed monitoring methods. By pooling resources, communities can collectively invest in these wearable devices, thereby enhancing their capacity to independently monitor and respond to environmental challenges, fostering a more sustainable and healthy living environment.

Wearable devices: A potential solution for environmental monitoring

Wearables, defined as compact electronic devices or wireless-enabled computers seamlessly integrated into everyday accessories, clothing, or gadgets, provide a valuable avenue for marginalized communities to manage their environmental health actively. Some iterations of these wearables, like micro-chips or smart tattoos, represent more invasive options. These wearable technologies are primarily designed for collecting, transmitting, and analyzing data typically gathered from human or animal bodies. They can encompass purely mechanical devices or sophisticated mechatronic systems, skillfully constructed using a combination of sensors, actuators, and computational components (8).

As per Gao et al. (9) wearable electronics refer to devices designed to be worn or attached to human skin for the continuous and close monitoring of an individual's activities, without causing interruption or restriction to the user's movements. Building on this definition, wearables can be succinctly described as electronic devices that are worn as accessories on the human body. They are equipped with integrated sensors to continuously track and display various personal metrics. These metrics often include daily physical activity, heart rate, and sleep patterns, monitored in real time. Common examples of such devices encompass smartwatches, smart glasses, wearable cameras, and virtual reality headsets. Each of these wearables offers unique functionalities and contributes to the growing utility of personal electronic monitoring in everyday life.

Compared to conventional devices, these flexible electronic devices are low in cost and power efficient in their consumption, allowing uninterrupted data acquisition over a long time (10). Wearable devices are on high demand because of its numerous advantages in health care monitoring, environmental and noise pollution, entertainment, communication, and many others. Also, due to their cost-effectiveness, wearable devices can serve as a means for marginalized communities to monitor their environment and assess the impact of pollution on their lives. This approach empowers them to resist decisions that affect their health and environment. By narrowing down the specific details and insights collected through these devices, individuals or communities invested in environmental health are better prepared to address concerns in both practical and political contexts (11).

Types of wearable devices

The surge in demand for wearable devices can be attributed to their multifaceted functionalities, applicable across various personal and industrial domains. Prominent examples of wearables include smartphones, smartwatches, fitness trackers, and smart glasses, each offering a unique set of features. Smartphones, primarily serving as communication tools through text messages and voice calls, also host a plethora of applications for mapping, weather forecasting, and monitoring daily steps and heart rate.

Smartwatches go beyond merely displaying time; they are instrumental in tracking overall wellness by monitoring daily movements, heart rate, blood pressure, and body temperature, among other metrics. Similarly, fitness trackers are not just limited to counting daily steps and distance traveled. They offer a comprehensive view of one's health by tracking sleep patterns, calculating total daily calorie burn, and continuously monitoring heart rate, thus contributing significantly to the personalized health monitoring landscape.

Other smart devices

- *Smart glasses:* Wearable devices equipped with features beyond traditional eyewear. These glasses typically incorporate a small computer or display module, enabling them to provide information directly to the wearer. The recording and shooting functions of smart glasses may violate others' privacy. However, as long as the purpose is clear and the monitor system is perfect, smart glasses will not become a threat to privacy but a practical life assistant and medical tool. Google, for example, already plans to introduce contact lenses with built-in sensors that can detect users' blood sugar levels.
- *Smart clothes and socks smart clothes:* They collect body data from users through fabric sensors and collection devices, which can be used to monitor users' exercise data and heat consumption. Also, there are smart baby clothes for infants to monitor their physical condition.
- *Smart shoes*: Smart sneakers mainly collect users' sports data to help users improve their sports plans better. In addition, some smart sneakers have new motion detection functions, such as Nike's FuelBand SE, which reminds users to stand up and take a move once in a while.
- *Smart earphones*: Smart headphones have new methods of applications, such as intelligent voice analysis and processing, which allow users to operate the equipment more conveniently using voice commands. In the future, it may be possible to integrate sensors directly into in-ear headphones to monitor heart rate, body temperature, and movement (12)

Evaluating health risks linked to toxic exposure remains a formidable challenge in the realm of environmental justice. Established connections between specific chemical exposures and certain health conditions are well-documented. However, quantifying exposure levels—including the concentration, duration, and appropriate measurement methods—continues to be a contentious and complex task. This complexity is further amplified by the difficulty of distinguishing these exposures from other concurrent environmental factors (13,14).

In the context of environmental justice and the potential role of wearable devices, it's crucial to understand the concept of marginalized communities and the root causes of disparities and inequalities in our society. Marginalization refers to a systematic process in which specific groups are excluded or pushed to the fringe of political and socioeconomic spheres. This relegation is often based on factors such as race, ethnicity, socioeconomic status, geographical location, religion, language, sexual identity, and disability status. Understanding this framework is essential for addressing and mitigating the environmental injustices these communities face (15).

Causes of disparity in marginalized communities

A striking example of systemic disparity can be seen in a 1984 report by Cerrell Associates, commissioned by the California Waste Management Board. This report candidly advised both industry and state authorities to strategically site waste incinerators in neighborhoods characterized by "lower socioeconomic" status. The rationale behind this recommendation was grounded in the perception that these communities would present a significantly reduced likelihood of political opposition, highlighting a calculated approach to exploiting socioeconomic vulnerabilities (16).

In a 1996 paper, Heiman and colleagues (17) discussed a notable example of environmental disparity. Their research revealed the existence of a major commercial hazardous waste management site at a landfill in Adams County, Colorado, and an incinerator in East Liverpool, Ohio. Both of these facilities were located in areas with predominantly Caucasian populations. In a striking contrast, the paper identified that three of the largest hazardous waste landfills, which accounted for over forty percent of the nation's total permitted commercial capacity for hazardous waste, were situated exclusively within two African-American communities (Emelle, Alabama, and Alsen, Louisiana) and one Hispanic community (Kettleman City, California). Remarkably, Kettleman City did not have its own waste management facility. This situation underscored a concerning pattern in environmental justice, highlighting how communities of color were disproportionately impacted by the placement of hazardous waste facilities (17).

Communities that have been historically marginalized continue to grapple with the stark realities of environmental injustice. These groups, frequently facing discrimination due to factors like race, economic status, gender, or disabilities, are often deprived of essential societal benefits and opportunities. This disparity is evident in their lack of access to adequate healthcare, education, and sanitation infrastructure, among other basic necessities (6). Significantly, Black communities and those living in lower socioeconomic conditions are the most vulnerable to environmental hazards, including air, water, soil, and noise pollution. The deep-seated causes of these environmental injustices are multifaceted and complex, as discussed in the following sections.

Historical inequities

Throughout American history, Black communities have faced persistent marginalization, a legacy that originates from the country's foundational years and its intricate history with slavery. The systemic racism, economic inequalities, and societal disparities that continue to impact Black communities today are deeply rooted in this period, where slavery was an entrenched institution in American society (18).

The legacy of slavery left an indelible mark on the development of the United States. Black people were subjected to unimaginable discrimination and the denial of fundamental rights. This tragic history laid the groundwork for the systemic racism that persists in various forms. Economic disparities have persisted as a consequence of centuries of unequal treatment, with Black individuals being deprived of opportunities and resources (19).

These historic injustices have contributed to a stark contrast in the exposure and health outcomes of Black communities when compared to other racial groups. The consequences of this deep-seated discrimination continue to be felt today, underscoring the need for ongoing efforts to address and rectify these disparities (20). In the history of the United States, minority communities have endured subpar educational systems, with even those fortunate enough to attend schools often facing bullying and discrimination based on their racial background. This unfortunate reality has led to a significant number of students dropping out of school, contributing to increased crime rates within these communities (21). These historical disadvantages have persisted over time, exacerbating the divide between marginalized communities and the rest of society, thus perpetuating social and economic disparities.

The roots of this systemic racism trace back to the country's early history. It began when enslaved Black individuals were denied basic human rights and were counted as only three-fifths of a person for the purpose of determining state representation in Congress. Even after the Emancipation Proclamation and the conclusion of the American Civil War, Black Americans still faced harsh restrictions through the imposition of Black Codes, which limited freedoms and compelled many to work for minimal or no wages (22).

The Civil Rights Act of 1866 was a landmark piece of legislation in the United States that affirmed the rights of Black people, particularly in matters related to property, labor, and contracts. However, it did not address voting rights or the ability to hold political office, which were issues later tackled by the 15th Amendment in 1870, granting Black men the right to vote. During the subsequent Jim Crow era, a range of segregationist policies were implemented, which had profound and lasting effects on the Black community. These policies entrenched poverty and denied Black Americans numerous economic and educational opportunities. Furthermore, in the 1930s, the discriminatory practice of redlining was instituted. This practice, carried out by federal housing agencies and private lenders, systematically denied financial services such as mortgages and insurance to residents in certain areas, predominantly those with a high concentration of Black residents. The impact of redlining was severe – it led to a decrease in property values in these areas, a deterioration in the quality of local schools and stores, and limited access to equitable healthcare, further exacerbating the socioeconomic challenges faced by the Black community (18).

Historically, communities of color in the United States have faced significant challenges in accessing their voting rights. These challenges were often rooted in systemic racism, which played a primary role in creating disparities in voter suppression. Various policies and practices, such as literacy tests, poll taxes, and other discriminatory measures, were explicitly designed to limit the voting rights of these communities. In contemporary times, there are concerns that certain policies and practices may continue to limit ballot access for communities of color. This includes issues like strict voter ID laws, reduction of early voting periods, and the closure of polling places in predominantly minority neighborhoods. Additionally, there is the phenomenon of survey misreporting. This occurs when voter turnout among communities of color is inaccurately reported in surveys, often showing higher rates of participation than actually occur. This misreporting can have significant implications. It may lead to a misunderstanding of the true extent of voter suppression and could potentially influence the development of policies and practices that inadvertently or deliberately continue to suppress the vote among these groups (23).

A system of racial segregation and discrimination, known as Jim Crow laws, was prevalent in the United States from the late 1800s to the mid-1960s. These laws, enacted by state and local governments, enforced racial segregation in public places, including schools, housing, and transportation. The Jim Crow era also extended to voting, employment, and other areas of life, systematically marginalizing African Americans. During this period, African Americans were systematically denied the right to vote through various means. These included literacy tests, poll taxes, and violent intimidation, all designed to disenfranchise them. These tactics effectively prevented African Americans from exercising their voting rights, which in turn allowed White politicians to maintain power and control over political and social institutions. The impact of these discriminatory practices contributed to the perpetuation of racial disparities and injustices that echoed into contemporary times, influencing policies and practices related to voting rights (24).

Zoning and land use policies

In their 1993 study, Massey and Denton (25) discussed how historical discrimination, ongoing inequality, and specific policies have contributed to racial segregation in housing in the United States. They highlight practices such as redlining, discriminatory lending, and exclusionary zoning as key factors. Their argument posits that 'systemic racism', rather than just individual preferences or market dynamics, plays a crucial role in creating disparities in housing access and quality for racial minorities. However, it's important to acknowledge that housing challenges are not exclusive to any single racial group. People living in poverty, irrespective of their race, often face significant difficulties related to housing. These include living in inadequate or unsafe conditions, struggling with high housing costs relative to their income, and facing the risk of homelessness. This broader perspective recognizes that while systemic racism significantly affects housing disparities, economic factors also play a critical role in housing challenges experienced by people across different communities (25).

Poor communities are often situated in areas that are redlined with less stringent zoning regulation making it easier for industries to locate there. The areas are marked as high risk, the people in such communities are denied financial services such as mortgages or loans to improve their lives. Also, because of the segregation the land regulations in these communities are not enforced to protect the people and the environment from pollution. Poor communities have become the dumping sites for most industrial toxic waste, landfill sites where garbage with different toxic contaminants are sited, waste incinerators which produce harmful chemicals to the environment are also found in these communities. These pollutants contaminate the air, soil and nearby water bodies.

This results in higher exposure to environmental hazards as the communities' experience air pollution by inhaling harmful gases which can lead to respiratory diseases. Their water is also polluted and by consuming the contaminated water many are at risk of suffering from waterborne diseases. The noise and chemicals from the industrialized factories set up in their locality adversely affect the people and environment. All this leads to the inhabitants of such communities being at higher risk of being diagnosed with respiratory diseases, lead and other contaminant poisoning, skin cancer, lung cancer, neurological issues, and cardiovascular diseases.

Economic factors

Oliver and Shapiro (26) asserted that 'systemic racism' is a primary driver of disparities in the wealth gap. They argue that the wealth gap between Black and White Americans is not simply the result of individual differences in savings or investment behavior but rather is the product of historical discrimination and inequality. They claim past policies such as redlining, discriminatory lending practices, and discriminatory employment practices contributed to the wealth gap (26).

Lower-income communities often lack the means to advocate effectively for enhancements in environmental conditions, quality healthcare, access to good education, and the implementation of rigorous land use regulations (27). This disparity is particularly pronounced within minority populations, where higher levels of education are less common, and many individuals find themselves in low-paying, menial jobs, directly impacting their overall quality of life. Regrettably, this reduced standard of living does not promote saving but tends to lead to the accumulation of debt, further diminishing their overall quality of life. These financial constraints frequently hinder their ability to secure mortgages and relocate to areas with superior environmental conditions (25). In addition to these challenges, discriminatory lending policies and high interest rates often contribute to the accumulation of debt, making it even more difficult for these communities to break the cycle of financial hardship.

Additionally, limited access to healthcare amplifies their vulnerability to environmental health risks, further compounding challenges (28) comprehensively explored the myriad factors contributing to wealth disparities, shedding light on a multifaceted and intricate challenge. Their research illuminated how income inequality, differences in homeownership rates, educational disparities, and variations in job opportunities all played crucial roles in shaping economic inequalities across various communities. These disparities were not confined to a single racial or ethnic group; they affected individuals from diverse backgrounds who were grappling with economic hardship. The disadvantages identified in their study extended to shared environmental challenges as well. These encompassed living in areas with poor air quality, contaminated water sources, proximity to toxic waste sites, labor market discrimination, and limited access to education and healthcare. Collectively, these adversities had a far-reaching impact, stretching across communities of all racial and ethnic backgrounds experiencing financial difficulties. It's important to underscore that despite the multifaceted nature of this issue, the literature consistently indicates that minority communities often bear a disproportionate burden (29). Their vulnerabilities, rooted in historical and ongoing systemic inequities, compound challenges, making it crucial to address these disparities comprehensively and systematically.

Limited political influence

The issue of underrepresentation of poor communities in mainstream media is a significant factor contributing to environmental justice challenges. Often, these communities are not adequately represented in the media, leading to a generalized lack of awareness and understanding of the specific adversities they face. This situation hampers their ability to effectively voice their concerns and needs, as highlighted in reference (24).

Furthermore, these communities typically wield less political clout, posing a substantial obstacle in advocating for and implementing policies that safeguard their interests. A recurring theme in environmental justice discourse is the inadequate representation of minority and impoverished communities in key decision-making forums. Their interests are often sidelined in environmental policy decisions, primarily because these communities seldom have representatives in influential governing bodies. This absence of representation means that decisions affecting their lives and environment are often made without their input or best interests in mind, leading to disproportionate exposure to environmental hazards and pollution. This systemic issue underscores the need for more inclusive representation in decision-making processes to address and rectify environmental injustices.

Proximity to industrial zones

Bullard (5) argued that communities of color are disproportionately burdened by environmental pollution and other environmental hazards. Policies such as zoning, land use, and environmental regulation have contributed to and perpetuate disparities, asserting that 'systemic racism' is a primary driver in environmental justice (5). Poor communities may be located closer to industrial zones because of lack of employment. The leaders in the local communities encourage industries to be set up in their locality to employ inhabitants of the community. Lack of political power in the poor communities encourages large factories that emit harmful chemical substances to be sited in these communities. They are exposed to these pollutants and their health is impacted negatively.

Lack of information and advocacy

People who have low health literacy may have difficulty understanding health information, navigating the healthcare system, and making informed decisions about their health (24). The majority of the population in marginalized communities are uneducated with little knowledge on environmental pollution and its risk on them. The people in the community are more interested in how to make ends meet instead of what is going on in their environment. These victims do not have any idea of the risk of exposure and its long-term effects on them. Also, they have less advocacy dedicated to their concerns because they lack representation. Their voices are barely heard, and the challenges of these vulnerable people are not considered as important and are totally ignored.

Wearable devices for environmental monitoring: Air quality monitoring

With an increase in industrialization in marginalized communities, it is very important to monitor the various air pollutants in the communities both indoors and outdoors. Exposure to air pollutants over a long period of time can have adverse effects of human beings and can cause respiratory diseases such as asthma and lung cancer. Air quality monitoring systems are very useful in effectively monitoring air pollution, allowing for active assessment of air pollutants to identify excess levels early. In the traditional context, air quality monitoring stations are typically characterized by their large size and high installation and maintenance costs. This restricts their potential for widespread deployment in densely populated urban areas (30). It is, therefore, necessary to empower marginalized communities on the importance of wearable devices to monitor the air quality of their surroundings. The wearable devices are less expensive, user-friendly, and do not require technical expertise compared to the traditional ones. Every household in marginalized communities should be encouraged to have a couple to access their environment. The utilization of affordable sensor technology for air pollution monitoring has advanced significantly over the past decade. These user-friendly devices are portable, low-maintenance, and have the capability to facilitate near real-time, continuous monitoring (31).

Wearable devices for environmental monitoring

Table 1 below summarizes examples of wearable devices and their uses to monitor air quality in communities (32).

Monitoring indoor air quality involves assessing the air composition within enclosed spaces like schools, offices, and homes. Several factors, including the concentration of different gaseous and particulate pollutants influence air quality. Insufficient ventilation may elevate indoor pollutant levels, as it fails to introduce adequate outdoor air to dilute emissions from indoor sources. Elevated temperature and humidity levels can also lead to higher concentrations of certain pollutants (33).

Monitoring outdoor air involves measuring the concentrations of different pollutants, including Ozone (O3), sulfur dioxide (SO2), nitrogen dioxide (NO2), carbon monoxide (CO) and particulate matter (PM) at specific locations (34).

Table 1. Wearable devices for air monitoring

Wearable Device	Uses	Price
TZOA	Measures PM10 and PM2.5, atmospheric pressure, humidity, temperature, ultraviolet exposure, and ambient light.	Less than $106
ATMOTUBE PRO	Measures PM1, PM2.5, and PM12, volatile organic compounds (VOC) in real-time, humidity, temperature, and atmospheric pressure.	Less than $370
ATMOTUBE PLUS	Measures pressure, temperature, humidity, and VOC.	Less than $53
THE WYND AIR QUALITY TRACKER	Senses airborne PM, including dust, allergens, and industrial pollution.	Uses iOS and Android application.
AIRBEAM	Monitors PM1, PM2.5, PM10, temperature, and humidity. Detects outdoor and indoor pollution.	Uses iOS and Android application. It also utilizes WiFi and cellular network.
HUMA	Measures CO_2, VOC, PM1, PM2.5, and PM10 in indoor environments. It also measures temperature and humidity.	

The concentration of atmospheric pollutants depends on the location, and therefore, also the time and space of the pollutant concentration are important to avoid dangerous exposures of humans (35). Depending on the location, the concentration of air particles may vary between different people in the same community. It is also important to note that paints, chemicals, detergents, behaviors such as smoking, and many others can change air quality, resulting in different homes in the same community.

A desirable approach is that air quality sensors are combined or communicated with other everyday portable devices (smartphones, tablets, and laptops) providing instantaneous and easily understandable information readings. An advantage for sensor development would be to contain as many contaminant detectors as possible at the same time, resulting in a challenge for most of the currently developed sensors and integrated platforms, due to the rapidly increasing size and complexity of both hardware and software instruments required to operate the different technologies (36).

It is worth noting that accumulating different data from the individuals in the community and trying to draw a conclusion from such data may be inaccurate due to many factors. Measuring atmospheric pollutants is challenging. Some of the difficulties in the analysis of air pollutants are their low concentration, complex chemical composition, and the presence of mixtures of compounds in the air. Standard monitoring devices applied to calculate pollutant exposure use a variety of measurement methods depending on the class of pollutants being measured. For instance, particulate matter concentrations are measured through gravimetric analysis and light-scattering devices. Light-scattering (LS) monitors use a laser beam to shine particles located in a chamber. A light detector then measures the scattered light which depends on the concentration and size of the particles; then, a constant air flow to feed particles into the chamber is required to produce reliable estimates (37).

After the protest of the Warren county (3) many marginalized communities have become involved in their communities and try to resist any suspicious illegal dumping of chemicals in the communities. Many individuals have found a need to involve themselves in the various researches in their communities to help them in decision making that will affect them. Throughout the United States and globally, residents are becoming more aware of the impact of pollution sources on their communities, recognizing that exposure to pollutants in their living, working, and recreational areas may pose health risks. Communities are increasingly seeking tools to document these exposures and address environmental health disparities. Currently, regulatory air monitoring systems often fail to assess neighborhood variations in air quality at a sufficiently detailed spatial scale. The proliferation of low-cost air pollution sensors has empowered citizen scientists to collect and utilize air quality data, enhancing their ability to characterize and comprehend the environmental conditions in their localities. Involving communities in science and research is crucial for advancing public health and fostering awareness regarding the sources of air pollution, exposure routes, and the links between contaminants and health outcomes (38).

Ultraviolet (UV) exposure sensors

UV is the radiation from the sun that reaches the earth, which helps in the production of vitamin D to strengthen and develop bones. However, excessive UV can negatively affect humans, causing skin cancer, skin aging, and many other harmful conditions.

Skin cancer stands out as the most prevalent form of cancer on a global scale. It is estimated that approximately 5 million adults received treatment for skin cancer annually in the United States between 2007 and 2011, incurring average treatment costs of $8.1 billion per year (39). As the incidence of skin cancer is growing rapidly, it has become one of the greatest threats to public health and has created a substantial economic burden for skin cancer treatment, particularly in countries like New Zealand, Australia, United States, United Kingdom and Germany (40). The increase of skin cancer is mainly because of the exposure to the sun. The most proactive and effective method of preventing skin cancer is to increase public education and awareness on this matter, and promote sun protection practices (41).

The purpose of wearable UV sensors is to measure personal UV exposure (both UVA and UVB) and provide useful information to users. Because the UVA and UVB intensities are usually not informative to the public, the measured UV is usually converted to UVI or UV dose with reference to the Minimal Erythema Dose (MED). Recent advances in miniaturized electronics and materials have enabled the successful development of wearable UV sensors. Based on photoreaction, they can be classified into photosensitive film-based or electronic integrated sensors. Upon their exposure to UVR, photosensitive film-based sensors undergo photodegradation, while the electronic sensors generate electrical current from incident photon energy. Dosimeter and radiometer are different names for such sensors, based on their measuring capabilities. The radiometer can measure instantaneous Ultraviolet Index (UVI) while the dosimeter can measure the cumulative UV dose. Photosensitive film-based sensors are designed to be dosimeters, whereas electronic sensors are often designed to be radiometers. Since the cumulative UV dose is the integral of the UV intensity with respect to time, time-stamped UV intensity measured by the electronic radiometer can also be processed to determine the cumulative dose. The following text will be divided into two main sections, (i) the photosensitive film-based UV dosimeters, and (ii) electronic integrated UV sensors (42).

Portable water quality sensors

Access to clean water stands as one of the critical resources essential for sustaining life, and the quality of drinking water significantly influences the well-being and health of individuals (43). Water is essential in life and the quality of water needs to be monitored, to ensure individuals are not consuming contaminated water.

Traditional ways of monitoring quality water are expensive. However, these methods are time-consuming (leading to delayed detection of and response to contaminants) and not very cost-effective. There is thus a need for more extensive and efficient monitoring methods (44).

Various methodologies have been utilized to monitor different contaminant parameters in water, encompassing electrochemical, physical, and optical sensing. Of these, electrochemical sensing is the preferred approach (45).

Electrochemical and biosensors provide a cost-effective method for concurrently monitoring water contaminant parameters through a multisensory patch, making them well-suited for online monitoring of extensive water bodies like reservoirs. Traditional glass-based sensors in electrochemical sensing have limitations for online monitoring, as their responses may be affected by varying pressure and temperature conditions. In contrast, electrochemical solid-state sensors utilizing metal–oxides (MOx), polymers, or carbon-based materials (employing thick/thin film technology) prove superior and are suitable for integration into wireless sensor networks (46).

Potentiometric and amperometric sensors

Among various sensor configurations, potentiometric sensors are extensively used to monitor pH and dissolved oxygen (DO). These electrochemical sensors, comprising sensitive and reference electrodes (REs), provide a straightforward and appealing approach, with their sensitivity assessed through the Nernstian equations (47).

Some sensors use a reference electrode (RE) made with a thick film of Ag/AgCl/KCl. These sensors show excellent stability over a long time, similar to glass reference electrodes. As a result, they work well for tasks that require collecting data for a long time (48).

Because it is really good at sensing things, stays stable, and lasts a long time, RuO2 is often used in pH and dissolved oxygen sensors. With RuO2, a pH sensor that measures from 2 to 13 (with a sensitivity of 58 mV/pH at 23°C) and a dissolved oxygen sensor that measures from 0.6 to 8.0 ppm log [O2] (from -4.71 to -3.59, with a sensitivity of -41 mV/decade at pH 8) have been made. These sensors work really well (49). The responsiveness of these sensors is notably affected by water temperature, displaying slower responses in colder conditions. For instance, at 9°C, the pH sensor exhibits a response time of 8–10 minutes compared to 1–2 seconds at higher temperatures (23°C) (50).

Silicon-based thin film sensors have found application in various contexts [52]. Their exceptional response consistency presents a promising Water Quality Monitoring (WQM) opportunity. However, a significant challenge associated with these sensors is the absence of compatible reference electrodes (REs). Numerous thin film-based Ag/AgCl REs studies have reported drift issues (51). To address this concern, a solid-state Ag/AgCl electrode can be situated in a miniature tank containing a KCl solution to enhance ion exchange, as demonstrated in the case of a nitrite monitoring sensor (52).

This sensor design holds promise for monitoring various analytes, including phosphates and ammonium. With further modifications to the working electrode (WE), there's potential to adapt this design for monitoring urea and ammonia. An array of RuO2-based sensitive electrodes (SE) has also been implemented to reduce measurement errors in microfabricated sensors developed using Ion-Sensitive Field-Effect Transistor (ISFET) technology (53). These sensors exhibit impressive performance with a sensitivity of 55.64 mV/pH and a low drift rate of 0.38 mV/h at pH. Such sensor arrays could be valuable for monitoring parameters like free chlorine, dissolved oxygen (DO), ions, and heavy metals (46).

Fixing problems with the reference electrode (RE) in potentiometric sensors means using the interdigitated electrode (IDE) design. This design is used in different types of sensors, like conductive, capacitive, impedance, and chemiresistive (two electrodes)-based sensors. Different materials, like metal–oxides, polymers, and carbon, work well with the electrodes in IDE-based sensors (54, 55). Among the notable IDE-based sensors documented for Water Quality Monitoring (WQM), hydrogel (polymer) stands out. This hydrogel exhibits both biocompatibility and cost-effectiveness in terms of materials and fabrication. The electrical properties of hydrogels, including conductivity, undergo changes upon interaction with analytes. (56, 57). The downsized pH sensor comprises an active electrode in the form of a hydrogel made from polypyrrole and polyaniline. However, notable limitations of the hydrogel-based sensor include its diminished mechanical strength and relatively short lifespan.

Interdigitated and chemiresistive-based sensors

Chemiresistive sensing represents another category of sensors that operates without the need for a reference electrode (RE). An example is the paper-based chemisistive sensor designed for the real-time monitoring of free chlorine (58). Utilizing a nanohybrid ink comprised of graphene and PEDOT: PSS, this sensor operates as a chemiresistive pH sensor. In another application, chemiresistive pH sensors, incorporating nanocomposites of single-wall carbon nanotubes (SWCNTs) and Nafion as the sensitive electrode (SE), have been investigated for Water Quality Monitoring (WQM). These sensors are employed in conjunction with drones equipped with wireless communication capabilities (59). The inclusion of a Nafion layer improves the functionality of the flexible sensor by mitigating the deterioration of electrical properties (60). The characteristics are affected by the cracking, and in some cases, breaking, of the sensitive electrode (SE) during bending. Additionally, findings from this sensor type indicate that sensitivity could be heightened by augmenting the number of printed SE layers. This same setup could be applied for real-time monitoring of conductivity, detection of chloride ions, and temperature sensing. Moreover, diverse forms of carbon nanotubes (CNTs) could be employed to enhance sensing performance (61). These electrochemical sensors are important to use in marginalized communities to monitor the water quality used by inhabitants. The sensors detect and measure the chemical components in the water available. The sensors provide real time information such as the pH, and dissolved ions to the user rather than depending on the government to provide findings of research over a period. Users of these electrochemical sensors which can promote water safety and detect contamination of water in marginalized communities.

Citizen-led water quality assessments

Citizen science, a burgeoning trend, has garnered significant popularity, particularly within the realms of ecology, biology, and environmental monitoring. This collaborative approach involves active engagement and contributions from members of the public, who, despite lacking formal scientific training, play pivotal roles in data collection, analysis, and decision-making processes. The inclusive nature of citizen science not only fosters a sense of community involvement but also broadens the scope and scale of scientific inquiry, enabling a diverse range of individuals to actively contribute to our understanding of the natural world (60). This encompasses the monitoring of water quality, including voluntary contributions to watershed health assessments within different programs in the United States, initiated subsequent to the implementation of the Clean Water Act in 1972 (62). Engagement in citizen science has the capacity to markedly extend data collection and analysis, accomplishing this at a fraction of the cost compared to conventional scientific campaigns (63). Education is a fundamental driver for engaging in citizen science, entailing the sharing of knowledge about the frameworks, assumptions, and intricacies that constitute the scientific process (64). Goals of increasing environmental awareness, promoting pro-environmental attitudes (65) and reconnecting people to nature (60) are often inherent within environmental citizen sciences (such as water quality monitoring), which have also been used to include citizens in policy-relevant science (66).

Citizen inexperience about how to best collect scientific data can indeed bias or skew data, hindering data quality and reliability (67). Thus, the challenge of understanding how non-professionals operate within scientific programs, including the resultant effect on data quality, has necessitated the development of citizen science frameworks and best practices for practitioners (66).

Despite evidence that citizen data can rival professional data, and a growing understanding of what constitutes 'good' citizen science, surveys of scientist perceptions show that concerns regarding data quality remain a significant barrier for trusting scientific conclusions derived from citizen science data (68)This mistrust is particularly concerning for policy-relevant science such as environmental research, where apprehension regarding data quality can hamper the use of results derived from citizen data in high-level policy and decision-making (62).

Further studies also question whether citizen science effectively engages citizens, such as within environmental policies or management controversies (69). To strengthen citizen led water quality in marginalized communities, the research team should partner with the different community leaders of the community understudy. Relationships can be established through face-to-face meetings, programs such as seminars, fairs and health forums. Through these processes, community leaders volunteer to participate encouraging other inhabitants to also get involved in the study. This encourages continuous support from the community.

Promoting access to safe drinking water

International human rights law mandates that nations strive for universal access to water and sanitation without discrimination, focusing on those in greatest need. The Committee on Economic, Social, and Cultural Rights, in its General Comment No 15, and the Special Rapporteur on the human right to safe drinking water provide essential guidelines for states in implementing these rights. Key elements include:

- *Availability:* Ensuring a sufficient and continuous water supply for personal and domestic uses, encompassing drinking, food preparation, clothes washing and personal and household hygiene. Adequate sanitation facilities must be available within or near each household, as well as in health or educational institutions, workplaces, and other public spaces to meet the needs of every individual.
- *Accessibility:* Making water and sanitation facilities physically accessible and within safe reach for all segments of the population, with consideration for specific groups such as persons with disabilities, women, children, and older persons.
- *Affordability:* Ensuring that water services are affordable for everyone, preventing any denial of access to safe drinking water based on financial constraints.
- *Quality and safety:* Guaranteeing that water for personal and domestic use is safe and free from micro-organisms, chemical substances, and radiological hazards that pose a threat to health.

Sanitation facilities must be hygienically safe, preventing contact with human excreta by humans, animals, or insects.
- *Acceptability:* Ensuring that all water and sanitation facilities are culturally acceptable and appropriate, taking into account gender, life-cycle, and privacy requirements.

Consumption of contaminated water can result in various illnesses, including cholera, hepatitis A, typhoid, and arsenic poisoning (70). Bacterial and viral pathogens, pathogenic protozoa, and other water-borne agents contribute to over five million deaths annually from water-borne diseases, leading to diarrhea and fluid/electrolyte loss (71).

VanDerslice stated (72) that many low income and minority communities did not have access to piped water. It is difficult to determine if a statistically significant relationship exists between income and access to water because many water systems do not collect demographic information from customers. However, this would still not include those relying on private drinking water systems. While a 2007 survey estimated that 0.5–1% of U.S. households lacked access to piped water, in some low income and minority areas, entire communities did not have piped water. In California, counties with a high percentage of minorities had a greater percentage of drinking water violations, 42% compared to 16% (72).

Many people in rural communities rely on private wells and/or natural springs for drinking water supply. Periodic testing for contaminants should be standard practice; however, the EPA (Environmental Protection Agency) does not regulate private wells and natural springs. The responsibility for scheduled testing falls to the homeowners, which could be a costly deterrent for low-income residents. Many people in these areas lack the means for regular water testing and may be consuming unsafe water. Boiling does not remove all harmful substances from the water, and contaminants may remain present in wells for years without the owner's knowledge (73).

Noise pollution monitors

Noise mapping serves as a visual depiction of the distribution of sound levels within a specific locale, offering an effective method for assessing noise in urban environments. Additionally, it aids in visually representing noise patterns in regions where land uses are particularly susceptible to noise. This contemporary approach to evaluating noise levels contributes to planning strategies aimed at mitigating the adverse effects of noise pollution (74).

The swift advancement of urbanization is resulting in notable levels of air and noise pollution. Consequently, extensive research endeavors are directed towards the development of detailed pollution and noise maps aimed at identifying urban areas causing significant adverse effects on human health. Conventional measurement techniques typically rely on costly and stationary equipment, rendering them unsuitable for the dynamic nature of urban environments due to the low spatio-temporal density of measurements. In contrast, the increasing ubiquity of mobile phones and their technological capabilities present a new avenue for citizen-assisted environmental monitoring.

A solution known as mobile crowdsensing (MCS) for monitoring air quality and noise pollution provides a practical illustration of a real-world system deployment, encompassing sensor calibration, data acquisition, and analysis. This approach reveals a correlation between elevated levels of air and noise pollution during peak hours, attributed to increased vehicular activity on the streets (75).

Monitoring noise using mobile phones

Smartphones offer a multitude of applications specifically crafted for measuring sound or evaluating noise levels. For instance, a search conducted on June 1, 2013, within the Apple AppStore using the keyword "sound meter" yielded 120 mobile applications compatible with iPhones. Broadening the search with terms like "noise" or "loudness" would extend this selection. Similarly, a comparable exploration in Android Market, Microsoft Mobile Marketplace, or Nokia Ovi might introduce an additional hundred mobile applications to the inventory (76).

Nevertheless, it's important to note that smartphones are not effortlessly and immediately deployable as sound meters to generate data for noise management. A significant portion of these mobile applications was primarily created for entertainment purposes, enabling users to gain a general understanding of the noise levels they encounter at specific locations and times, albeit without a high degree of accuracy (76).

An examination of scientific literature revealed only three mobile phone applications that were meticulously designed, implemented, and tested for measuring noise through mobile phones within a framework promoting community participation. One notable example is NoiseTube, which was developed in 2009 by a collaborative effort involving European universities from France, Belgium and the Netherlands (77). Another application, known as NoiseSpy, was crafted in 2010 by the University of Cambridge in United Kingdom, as outlined by Kanjo in 2010. Additionally, the Ear-Phone, which emerged in 2010, was spearheaded by the University of New South Wales and CSIRO in Australia, with collaboration from Portland State University in the United States (78, 79). These serve as three recent examples that align with the research presented in this context. The NoiseTube project aimed to establish a participatory network for monitoring noise pollution, allowing both citizens and governmental bodies to comprehend the issue of urban noise pollution and its societal repercussions. This initiative was prompted by the European Noise Directive (END), which emphasized creating noise maps to comprehensively depict the population's noise exposure. In a laboratory experiment comparing NoiseTube to a scientific sound meter, the precision achieved was +4 dB within a sound scale ranging from 35 to 100 dB.

In 2012, there was a real-world test of NoiseTube within a participatory context, as outlined by D'Hondt, Stevens et al. (80) in 2013. The objective was to demonstrate that, if appropriately executed, participatory techniques can attain accuracy levels equivalent to those demanded by conventional noise mapping methods.

Much like the earlier mobile phone application, NoiseSpy functions as a sound sensing system that transforms a mobile phone into an affordable data logger for tracking environmental noise. This enables users to explore urban areas while collectively visualizing noise levels. The primary goal of NoiseSpy was to highlight the mobile phone application's potential for involving people in widespread participation in environmental campaigns, thereby raising awareness of environmental issues and supporting educational initiatives. The utilization of the data for planning and management appears to be of secondary importance, as no assessment of the data's accuracy has been reported (76).

The Ear-Phone project aimed to create noise maps, considering the inherent challenges posed by data provision from citizens and mobile phones, such as the fragmented and incomplete nature of data in both space and time. The Ear-Phone project devised a methodology based on compressive sensing to address the issue of reconstructing noise maps from incomplete and random samples gathered through crowd-sourced data collection. In field tests conducted by researchers, Ear-Phone exhibited a precision of +2.7 dB when compared to commercial sound meters.

Results from a case study involving six participants indicated that using data from only one person did not reveal distinct patterns in the reconstruction. However, incorporating data from multiple individuals gradually exposed differences between noisy and quiet areas. Moreover, beyond a certain threshold, increasing the number of data contributors did not significantly enhance the accuracy of the reconstruction. This method and experiment underscore the significance of widespread participation in citizen science (76).

Health monitoring for environmental justice

A growing body of evidence indicates that low-income groups, a disproportionate percentage of which are people of color, tend to be both more exposed to many environmental pollutants as well as more susceptible to related health effects than the general population. Even though there is not enough statistical evidence to proof, many observational studies conducted found that people of color, people of low income live close to dumping sites, reside in urban areas where ambient levels of many air pollutants tend to be higher, eat significantly greater amounts of contaminated fish, and be employed in potentially dangerous occupations. It is known that their minority communities are more exposed to environmental hazards and suffer adversely from disabilities, diseases such as skin cancers, kidney problems and more (81).

The role of wearable devices in health tracking

Diabetes is a global persistent health condition. Problems associated with diabetes incudes stroke, blindness, heart diseases which can in the long term lead to death. Report provided by the World Health Organization, diabetes is on the rise and diabetic patients has increased from 108 million in 1980 to 422 million in 2014 implying that about 8.5% of adults aged 18 years and older had diabetes, with a potential to surpass 500 million cases in 2030 (82).

Type 1 diabetes (T1D) is caused by insufficient insulin secretion by the pancreas, it can be managed by dispensing insulin. Type 2 diabetes (T2D), caused by bad daily habits, e.g., physical inactivity and unhealthy diet (83).

It is essential to properly manage diabetic patients to reduce the risk of complications. This management can be done by monitoring the glucose levels in a patient's blood. Diabetic patients also need constant monitoring of their diet, exercise, taking medications and injecting insulin and therefore the need to use the right sensors (84). Lately, BG monitoring has been transformed by the enhancement of Continuous Glucose Monitoring (CGM) sensors, that measure glucose concentration almost without interruption (1–5 min sampling period) for days (85). Low impact needle sensor is used by these equipments fixed in the subcutaneous tissue, in the abdomen or on the arm which measures an electrical current signal generated by the glucose-oxidase reaction.

Air quality and diabetes

The main causes of diabetes are known to be poor lifestyle, unhealthy diet, lack of exercise and genetic background. With the increase in the rise of diabetes among children and adults worldwide, attention has been drawn to the fact that exposure of environmental pollutants contributes to the prevalence of diabetes (86). Various studies confirms that pollutants can disrupt glucose homeostasis and promote metabolic dysfunction (87). Occasional use of pesticides and chemicals found in homes such as flame retardants and bisphenol have been associated with metabolic dysfunction (88). According to research conducted by Jagai et al. (86), it was concluded that air quality in sparsely populated and less urbanized areas has a impact on the prevalence of diabetes. Additionally, environmental pollutants associated with diabetes have been shown to disproportionately affect minority communities (89). Diabetes unevenly impacts African Americans, Latinos, and low-income individuals. In contrast to non-Hispanics, the possibility of developing diabetes is projected to be 66% higher for Hispanics and 77% more for the black race (90).

Several studies have indicated elevated exposure to diabetogenic endocrine-disrupting chemicals (EDCs), including polychlorinated biphenyls, organochlorine pesticides, multiple chemical constituents of air pollution, bisphenol A, and phthalates has been a major cause of prevalence of diabetes among the black race and low-income communities (89). EDC is defined as a chemical or mixture of chemicals that disrupts with any aspect of hormone action (91). EDCs can disrupt insulin secretion and function along with affecting other ways that regulate glucose homeostasis (91). PCB is also another substance that can elevate diabetes among the black race. Among female residents of Anniston, serum PCB levels were significantly associated with diabetes (92). Another toxic chemical increasing the rate of diabetes in the minority communities is the organochlorine (OC) pesticide. This particular chemical was banned but however there are still traces found in marginalized communities.

We also know for a fact metal such as zinc, iron manganese are needed by humans, metals such as lead and mercury are harmful to humans. Exposure of humans to lead and mercury can be a factor in the prevalence of diabetes amongst humans. Even though lead exposure has reduced in recent years in the developed countries, inhabitants of poor communities are still exposed to lead (93). A typical example is the incident at Flint in Michigan, there was an exposure of lead in the water system of the community which was a water source to the majority of the population (94). It is important to note that exposure to lead only cannot be the cause to diabetes, but other factors including lead exposure makes one at risk of being diabetic. The exposure of metals such as lead to individuals, leads to induce oxidative stress in biological systems. This holds significance since numerous crucial elements of the insulin signaling pathway are known to be constrained by reactive oxygen specific (ROS), fostering the growth of insulin obstruction and diabetes (95). Recent studies have shown a significant relationship between blood lead levels and indicators of oxidative stress in the population. Findings suggest that oxidative stress should be considered in the progression of lead related diseases, even amongst individuals with relatively low exposure to lead (i.e., <10 μg/dL) (96). Most of biological samples ofT2D patients exhibit traces of toxic metals indicating exposure to harmful metals such as lead and nickel. Some of the toxic metals can interfere with the glucose uptake and alter the related molecular mechanism in glucose regulation (97).

Cardiovascular health monitoring

Wearable heart rate monitors are used to monitor the heart rate (HR) of individuals and provide valuable information such as cardiovascular health, duration of exercise, sleep pattern and steps taken (98). Traditional methods of recording HR are more expensive and require software which are used in medical or research laboratories, wearable devices are used to measure HR of individuals because they are less expensive, readily available and have a friendly interface to use (98). Wearable devices used for monitoring heart rates includes the bracelet-sized trackers like the Basis Carbon Steel, the Samsung Gear Fit, Apple watch and the Withings Pulse O2 tout which sometimes runs on applications such as Androids or IOS. Devices such as the Apple Watch, Samsung Galaxy Gear 2, and Samsung Galaxy S5 mobile phone include embedded heart rate monitors (99), they use photoplethysmogram (PPG) for the measurement of HR of individuals (100). They use light to track your blood and through that the heart rate is measured. These devices illuminate the capillaries with a sensor that gauges rates at which the blood pumps (99). By illuminating your capillaries with a light emitting diode (LED), a sensor adjacent to the light measures the frequency at which your blood pumps your heart rate. These devices are inexpensive and simple to measure the HR of people but its accuracy is questionned. It also vulnerable to motion-induced noise, meaning the optical sensor in these devices expect the user not to move but be still, no talking and even sweating Also using these bracelet sized trackers is not always accurate and does not always give the true heart rate. This because by the time blood reaches the capillaries in your wrist, it has already reduced to a rate which is not the actual heart rate. We also have the Garmin Vivofit which is a chest strap heart rate monitor which is more preferred because it functions like the electrocardiogram (EKG) by measuring electrical pulse (beats per minute) reading. The readings on these devices are more accurate because heart rate monitor is used in conjugation with the trackers (99). However, it cannot read accelerated heart rates after exercises or workouts but it is accurate for measuring HR both at rest and moderate exercises (101). This device has improved signal-to-noise ratio (SNR) meaning it can tolerate noise and movement better than wrist worn devices. It also has high transmittance in the visible light spectrum, it is waterproof and can withstand sweat, it is of a high quality and therefore can last long (102).

Impact of environmental factors on cardiovascular health

Cardiovascular disease (CVD) is a leading cause of death worldwide. CVD was a major cause of death for an estimated 13 million people globally in 2010, a quarter of the global totally (increased from just one in five deaths 20 years earlier) (103). Many factors account for the prevalence of CVD, conditions like diabetes, obesity and, behaviors like unhealthy diet, physical inactivity, and too much alcohol can increase a person's risk of heart disease

(105). The major cause of environmental pollution is air pollution, then water and soil pollution with pesticides and other chemicals. Other factors such light exposure, noise from traffic and climate change can negatively impact individual health and can cause CVD (106).

Environmental exposure to certain chemicals and metals can increase the risk of one developing CVD. According to World Health Organization (WHO), exposure to metals such as lead, calcium and arsenic can cause people to develop CVD (107). Vehicle emission, burning of trees, tire fragmentation, dust and industrial combustion releases gases such carbon monoxide (CO), oxides of nitrogen, sulfur dioxide (SO2), ozone, lead are released directly into the air. This causes air pollution leading to the prevalence of CVD globally (108). Long-term exposure to particulate matter is a major cause to CVD leading to death with the largest effects due to ischemic heart disease (108).

A good soil is needed for the cultivation of crops for human survival, the soil is needed to absorb carbon which reduces climate change. Soil stores water and protects waterways, thus preventing floods and waterborne diseases. Deposit of toxic waste, pesticides, heavy metals, deforestation on the soil contaminates the soil increase risk of cardiovascular diseases on the population (109). "While these pollutants differ in their chemical composition, they cause disease through shared pathophysiological pathways centered on oxidative stress and inflammation leading to a dysregulation of circadian rhythms. Oxidative stress and inflammation in response to contamination with plastic, heavy metals, overfertilization, pesticides, and toxic agents represent major pathophysiologic mechanisms causing cardiovascular, neurodegenerative, and metabolic diseases" (109).

Built environment is the physical changes and construction made by man on the natural environment and surroundings. It includes building or structures as shelter, streets, shaping spaces meeting places, landmarks. Certain elements of structures such as doors, windows, walls, floors, rooms sizes and function make up the built environment (110). Built environments comprises of buildings, spaces around buildings, layout of communities, transportation infrastructure, and parks designed by humans for interaction (111). Built environment in modern cities is a major factor of obesity and hypertension (112). Physical inactivity is a common attribute of the lives of people living in built environment. Labour saving devices are used for household chores, remote jobs causing people to work from home and easy access to individual cars have discouraged people from moving and walking as a means of transportation. Between 1977 and 1995, the number of all walking trips decreased by 32% for adults, with similar reductions for youth (113). People become active with the use of public transportation and they are less likely to be overweight and obese than people who do not use public transportation (114). Because of built of environment there is easy access to groceries and eateries which encourages eating of junk food amongst individual with little or no physical activity. Through these societal changes, chronic diseases and CVD have people become prevalent amongst the working force (115). To minimize cardiovascular disease and death, cities need planning by encouraging the use of more buses than individuals driving, developing greener communities, tree planting to make our environment safe (116).

Challenges and considerations

From the paper it is important to note that wearable devices are very important in our everyday life and is demand is on the rise because of its various functionalities. However, it has key challenges such as data privacy and security concerns, technological accessibility, accuracy, and validation especially in environmental monitoring which needs to be addressed.

Data privacy and security concerns

Wearable devices use personal data for its set-up. Users share personal details such as name, date of birth, phone number, address, biometric features and bank account to create profiles. The political preference race, religious denominations and location of individuals are easily captured making it easy to identify individuals (117). Many users of these wearable devices are not aware of the privacy risk associated with the use of these devices. Wearable devices have in built sensors that can give personal information of the user such as location, physiological and emotional behaviors to a third party (118). Wearable devices functions by the use of the internet, this could lead leakage of information based on interaction among devices even though they may not be related (119). Wearable devices are connected to applications using Wifi and Bluetooth which makes the user vulnerable to cyber security threats causing huge lost to individuals and companies (117). Many users have false sense of privacy meaning as they think that wearable devices take right measures to protect user's sensitive information. They also believe that since they are not using keyboards on the wearables they are not entering or any sensitive information. Users also are not aware of kind of data is taken and stored by these wearable devices (120). Data and activity of users of wearable devices are systematically captured and sold to third party marketing companies. The activities of users can easily be traced and identified through videos, pictures, Global Position System (GPS) without the permission and consent of users. Even though this may not cause any harm to the users it is a breach of privacy (117).

Technological accessibility and the digital divide

Even though wearables have become a necessity and are of high demand globally, these wearables still present challenges to users with disabilities. Most of these devices are not easily accessible and user friendly to the disabled (121). Manufacturers of these devices do not consider the requirements of the disabled people when creating applications for these devices. Because of their special needs, the wearable devices should have easy systems put in place to help the disabled to use the devices without any hindrance (121).

Wearable devices are very helpful and can be used by the older generation to monitor their heart rates, track their daily movements, and predict any unusual pattern in the user. However the older population also have difficulty in learning and using these devices. Many of them oppose change and the use of technological devices since they did not grow up with this kind of lifestyle (122). The older population find it difficult to personalize these devices by giving out their personal information (123).

Those who are economically stable have the purchasing power to buy these wearable devices than those living in marginalized communities. They can easily purchase the smart watches, heart rate monitors and even different brands of these (124). Those who can even purchase these devices in marginalized communities have limited access to pre-owned devices. Even though the majority of the low-income people use internet, their access is limited and unstable causing connectivity issues (125). High income communities have pay more for internet service and get the best services whiles many of those in the redlined communities have access to internet through their cellular devices and even those who may internet access at home have the poor services (126). It is also easier for the rich to maintain these devices when they get spoilt are simply replace them but the people in the marginalized communities may not even purchase a new one when their devices break down.

Environmental data accuracy and validity

Wearable devices are often created for its technological use without considering the society, culture and environmental policies they function within. The design of these devices should factor the society, culture and environmental policies (127). Wearable devices used for measuring the environment are mostly concerned with the indoor factors than outdoor factors. The use of wearable devices to monitor the outdoor mostly involves a combination of devices to get the accurate measurement of the environmental condition. To get a more accurate result, there needs to be a relationship between monitored data with data obtained through calibrated sensors of a reference instrument. Researchers analyze the data obtained but do not participate in the measuring of the environmental factors. This does not give a reflection of the exact variable being measured (31). To get accurate results using a wearable device, several devices need to be tested to select one that is suitable for the study. Access to data, accuracy and validation of data are some of the factors that will be considered before conducting the study which can be a constraint and cause a delay in the study (128). Many of the wearable devices may need some of technical key or permission before it can be used which can affect the accuracy of results because most of the users of these wearable devices from the marginalized communities have no limited experience on the usage (129). Another challenge is that wearable devices are not sturdy enough as the laboratory-based studies. They are not authenticated enough to be used in different spans of environmental conditions with different ranges in altitude, temperature and humidity levels (130).

Ethical considerations in environmental monitoring

Data obtained from wearable devices improves with data obtained from environmental sensors. The outcome received from wearables can be enhanced using different sensors to ascertain the type and impact of operation of users in a defined environment. To improve the lives of inhabitants in communities, it is better to observe possible causes of environmental conditions from a distance rather than depending on data provided by individual with the use of wearable devices (131). According to UNICEF, wearables are not designed with the user, that is, it does not generate tailor made solutions based on the needs and preference of the user. Manufacturers of wearables do not ensure solutions are considerate and beneficial especially to the marginalized communities. Wearables also suffer being scalable. They cannot be implemented in the various environments and communities in the ecosystem. Wearable devices are not designed to be replicable and adaptable across various countries and continents. Wearables for environmental measuring are not user friendly and are also difficult to maintain. UNICEF also stated that these devices are not data driven, they are not developed based on projects to measure milestones and track environment's progress effectively. Some wearable devices are expensive and cannot be purchased by the ordinary citizen. Wearables run on power, and in communities with power issues, wearable devices are not effective to use.

Future directions and recommendations

Wearable sensors provide large magnitude of data which enables detailed analysis, offering valuable insights into different aspects of users' health, activity, and behavior. Machine learning is an important tool that is needed to identify patterns, examine data for recurring trends and relationships to create meaningful insights. Machine learning will use intuitive steps rather than a systematic approach to determine different trends which are distinct to every user.

To use machine learning data obtained from the wearable sensor devices can provide can be stored a cloud computing platform and analyzed using machine learning tools. Machine learning can be integrated into the application of smartphones.

Machine learning provides precise analysis of the data of the user recognizing the diverse movement pattern for more comprehensive and accurate analysis (132).

Building awareness and digital literacy

Wearable technology is advancing quickly and rapidly, product development cycles can outpace testing, leading to upgraded products even before the product is comprehensively tested (133). The prevalence of wearable devices has necessitated for digital literacy to help effectively communicate with new technologies. In recent years, industries such as Google, Amazon, Facebook have scheduled announcements on the emergence of wearable and immersive technologies in transforming consumer markets and businesses (134). Acknowledging the anticipated outcomes of the new technologies, the 115th United States Congress created the Congressional Caucus on Virtual, Augmented and Mixed Reality Technologies in anticipation of the "tremendous potential for innovation in the fields of entertainment, education and healthcare" (134). Even though teaching digital technologies will become obsolete after some years, it is imperative to use teaching approaches that equips students for 21st century communications and for their future employment (135). Digital literacy can be enhanced through a collaboration with community libraries to provide programs and workshops on technological skills such us using emails, surfing on the internet(136). Libraries can engage people by providing training to new technologies such as artificial intelligence, robotics and 3D modeling (136).

Promoting ethical data collection and sharing

To promote ethical data collection and sharing we can promote a logical border which enables anonymous user identification to maintain privacy and security in digital systems. This will use a unique identification that does not expose personal details of the user. This process can be enhanced by setting up default user account which has inbuilt logical borders that restricts engagement to the minimum level (119). To reduce problems with data privacy and security concerns will be to introduce block chain technology. This is a structure that securely records and validates transactions across computer networks. The structure utilizes natural language processing to guarantee adherence with privacy and security policies that are permitted to be stored on the block chain which cannot be interfered with (137). The use of wearables has rapidly increase in society because of its importance in communication, however it still lacks compatibility on rules and regulations for a seamless function (127). The first step is to have it in design elements that is all inclusive of the semblance, individual responses and social influences. (138). The future innovation should include how a user's personal identification can be altered with the advancement of wearable devices.

Wearables should be designed to support the abilities of individuals especially those with disabilities, helping them to perform activities they find challenging to perform without any difficulty. This will help all individuals to build their identification and change them based on their conditions. Wearables becomes all-inclusive and accessible to everyone in society (127). Stakeholders be it private, public or individuals should intentionally be involved in the designing of these devices and in the governance framework to ensure that the finished product is an innovation of the old product which is functional to a large population. It prevents it from being under-utilized for the population it was manufactured for (138). There should be policy development clearly stating the goals, measurable outcomes and expected outcomes. Users should be educated of the effects of using wearable devices and methods of managing and retaining control of wearable devices to inform the users the kind of data is taken and stored by these wearable devices (138).

Strengthening community partnerships

To strengthen community partnerships, research teams should partner with the different community leaders of the community understudy. Relationships can be established through face-to-face meetings, programs such as seminars, fairs and health forums. Through these processes, community leaders volunteer to participate encouraging other inhabitants to also get involved in the study. This encourages continuous support from the community.

Conclusion

In conclusion, this paper has comprehensively explored the transformative potential of wearable devices in environmental justice and public health monitoring. Through detailed analysis of various sensor technologies, including air quality monitors, UV exposure sensors, and water quality sensors, we've established the critical role these devices play in empowering marginalized communities to actively engage in environmental health monitoring.

The paper demonstrates how wearable technology offers a unique opportunity for real-time data collection and personalized health management, particularly in communities disproportionately affected by environmental hazards. These technologies not only enhance individual awareness of environmental risks but also provide valuable data that can inform policy decisions and public health interventions.

Looking forward, the integration of advanced technologies such as AI and machine learning will further enhance the capabilities of these wearables, offering even more nuanced and accurate data analysis. However, challenges related to data privacy, security, and technological accessibility must be addressed to ensure these innovations benefit all segments of society equitably.

As we continue to grapple with the complex interplay of environmental factors and public health, wearable devices stand out as powerful tools in the pursuit of environmental justice. By bridging the gap between communities and technology, these devices not only empower individuals with crucial health data but also contribute significantly to our collective understanding and management of environmental health risks.

Acknowledgments

Conceptualization, E.O.-G.; methodology, A.M. and E.O.-G.; formal analysis, A.M.; investigation, A.M. and E.O.-G.; resources, E.O.-G.; data curation, A.M.; writing—original draft preparation, A.A.; writing—review and editing, A.M. and E.O.-G.; supervision, E.O.-G.; project administration, E.O.-G.; funding acquisition, E.O.-G. Funding Research reported in this publication was supported by the National Institute of General Medical Sciences of the National Institutes of Health under Award Number R16GM149473. The content is solely the responsibility of the authors and does not necessarily represent the official views of the National Institutes of Health. Conflicts of interest: The authors declare no conflict of interest.

References

[1] Pellow DN. What is critical environmental justice? New York: John Wiley Sons, 2017.
[2] Bullard RD, Mohai P, Saha R, Wright B. Toxic wastes and race at twenty: Why race still matters after all of these years. Environ Law 2008;38(2):371-411.
[3] Bullard RD. Ecological inequities and the new South: Black communities under siege. J Ethn Stud 1990;17(4):101-15.
[4] McGurty E. Transforming environmentalism: Warren County, PCBs, and the origins of environmental justice. New Brunswick, NJ: Rutgers University Press, 2009.
[5] Bullard RD. Confronting environmental racism: Voices from the grassroots. Boston, MA: South End Press, 1993.
[6] Pellow DN. Toward a critical environmental justice studies: Black Lives Matter as an environmental justice challenge. Du Bois review. Soc Sci Res Race 2016;13(2):221-36.
[7] Banzhaf S, Ma L, Timmins C. Environmental justice: The economics of race, place, and pollution. J Econ Perspect 2019;33(1):185-208.
[8] Nahavandi D, Alizadehsani R, Khosravi A, Acharya UR. Application of artificial intelligence in wearable devices: Opportunities and challenges. Comput Methods Programs Biomed 2022;213:106541.
[9] Gao W, Emaminejad S, Nyein HYY, Challa S, Chen K, Peck A, et al. Fully integrated wearable sensor arrays for multiplexed in situ perspiration analysis. Nature 2016;529(7587):509-14.
[10] Iqbal SM, Mahgoub I, Du E, Leavitt MA, Asghar W. Advances in healthcare wearable devices. NPJ Flexible Electronics 2021;5(1):9.
[11] Kane F, Abbate J, Landahl EC, Potosnak MJ. Monitoring particulate matter with wearable sensors and the influence on student environmental attitudes. Sensors 2022;22(3):1295.
[12] Jin CY, ed. A review of AI technologies for wearable devices. IOP Conference Series: Materials Science and Engineering, 2019.
[13] Tesh SN. Uncertain hazards: Environmental activists and scientific proof. Ithaca, NY: Cornell University Press, 2000.
[14] Vrijheid M. Health effects of residence near hazardous waste landfill sites: a review of epidemiologic literature. Environ Health Perspect 2000;108(suppl 1):101-12.
[15] Newman PA, Reid L, Tepjan S, Fantus S, Allan K, Nyoni T, et al. COVID-19 vaccine hesitancy among marginalized populations in the US and Canada: Protocol for a scoping review. PLoS One 2022;17(3):e0266120.
[16] Faber D. Capitalizing on environmental injustice: The polluter-industrial complex in the age of globalization. Lanham, MD: Rowman Littlefield, 2008.
[17] Heiman MK. Race, waste, and class: New perspectives on environmental justice. Antipode 1996;28(2):111-21.
[18] Churchwell K, Elkind MS, Benjamin RM, Carson AP, Chang EK, Lawrence W, et al. Call to action: structural racism as a fundamental driver of health disparities:

a presidential advisory from the American Heart Association. Circulation 2020;142(24):e454-68.
[19] Solomon D, Maxwell C, Castro A. Systemic inequality: Displacement, exclusion, and segregation. Washington, DC: Center for American Progress 2019;7.
[20] Williams DR, Mohammed SA, Leavell J, Collins C. Race, socioeconomic status, and health: complexities, ongoing challenges, and research opportunities. Anna NY Acad Sci 2010;1186(1):69-101.
[21] Childress S, Elmore R, Grossman A. How to manage urban school districts. Harvard Business Rev 2006;84(11):55.
[22] Reich SA. A working people: A history of African American workers since emancipation. Lanham, MD: Rowman Littlefield, 2013.
[23] Ansolabehere S, Hersh E. Validation: What big data reveal about survey misreporting and the real electorate. Political Anal 2012;20(4):437-59.
[24] Baker B. Systemic poverty, not systemic racism: An ethnography, analysis and critique. J Bus Divers 2023;23(2):1-25.
[25] Massey DS, Denton NA. American apartheid: Segregation and the making of the underclass. In: Grusky D, ed. Social stratification, class, race, and gender in sociological perspective, second edition. New York: Routledge; 2019:660-70.
[26] Oliver M, Shapiro T. Black wealth/white wealth: A new perspective on racial inequality. New York: Routledge, 2013.
[27] Baron SL, Beard S, Davis LK, Delp L, Forst L, Kidd-Taylor A, et al. Promoting integrated approaches to reducing health inequities among low-income workers: Applying a social ecological framework. Am J Ind Med 2014;57(5):539-56.
[28] Zou W, Lo D, Kochhar PS, Le XBD, Xia X, Feng Y, et al. Smart contract development: Challenges and opportunities. IEEE Trans Softw Eng 2019; 47(10):2084-106.
[29] Chong D, Kim D. The experiences and effects of economic status among racial and ethnic minorities. Am Polit Sci Rev 2006;100(3):335-51.
[30] Zheng K, Zhao S, Yang Z, Xiong X, Xiang W. Design and implementation of LPWA-based air quality monitoring system. IEEE Access 2016;4:3238-45.
[31] Salamone F, Masullo M, Sibilio S. Wearable devices for environmental monitoring in the built environment: A systematic review. Sensors 2021;21(14):4727.
[32] Bernasconi S, Angelucci A, Aliverti A. A scoping review on wearable devices for environmental monitoring and their application for health and wellness. Sensors 2022;22(16):5994.
[33] Bhattacharya S, Sridevi S, Pitchiah R, editors. Indoor air quality monitoring using wireless sensor network. In: 2012 Sixth International Conference on Sensing Technology (ICST), IEEE, 2012.
[34] Kumar P, Morawska L, Birmili W, Paasonen P, Hu M, Kulmala M, et al. Ultrafine particles in cities. Environ Int 2014;66:1-10.
[35] Elminir HK. Dependence of urban air pollutants on meteorology. Sci Total Environ 2005;350(1-3):225-37.

[36] Oluwasanya PW, Alzahrani A, Kumar V, Samad YA, Occhipinti LG. Portable multi-sensor air quality monitoring platform for personal exposure studies. IEEE Instrum Meas Mag 2019;22(5):36-44.
[37] Wang X, Chancellor G, Evenstad J, Farnsworth JE, Hase A, Olson GM, et al. A novel optical instrument for estimating size segregated aerosol mass concentration in real time. Aerosol Sci Technol 2009;43(9):939-50.
[38] Sai KBK, Mukherjee S, Sultana HP. Low cost IoT based air quality monitoring setup using arduino and MQ series sensors with dataset analysis. Procedia Comput Sci 2019;165:322-7.
[39] Guy Jr GP, Machlin SR, Ekwueme DU, Yabroff KR. Prevalence and costs of skin cancer treatment in the US, 2002− 2006 and 2007− 2011. Am J Prev Med 2015;48(2):183-7.
[40] Gordon LG, Rowell D. Health system costs of skin cancer and cost-effectiveness of skin cancer prevention and screening. Eur J Cancer Prev 2015;24(2):141-9.
[41] Armstrong BK, Kricker A, English DR. Sun exposure and skin cancer. Australas J Dermatol 1997;38:147-56.
[42] Huang X, Chalmers AN. Review of wearable and portable sensors for monitoring personal solar UV exposure. Ann Biomed Eng 2021;49:964-78.
[43] World Health Organization. Guidelines for drinking-water quality. Geneva: World Health Organization, 2004.
[44] Lambrou TP, Anastasiou CC, Panayiotou CG, Polycarpou MM. A low-cost sensor network for real-time monitoring and contamination detection in drinking water distribution systems. IEEE Sens J 2014;14(8):2765-72.
[45] Seymour I, O'Sullivan B, Lovera P, Rohan JF, O'Riordan A. Electrochemical detection of free-chlorine in water samples facilitated by in-situ pH control using interdigitated microelectrodes. Sens Actuators B Chem 2020;325:128774.
[46] Manjakkal L, Mitra S, Petillot YR, Shutler J, Scott EM, Willander M, et al. Connected sensors, innovative sensor deployment, and intelligent data analysis for online water quality monitoring. IEEE Internet Things J 2021;8(18):13805-24.
[47] Manjakkal L, Synkiewicz B, Zaraska K, Cvejin K, Kulawik J, Szwagierczak D. Development and characterization of miniaturized LTCC pH sensors with RuO2 based sensing electrodes. Sens Actuators B Chem 2016;223:641-9.
[48] Manjakkal L, Cvejin K, Kulawik J, Zaraska K, Szwagierczak D, Socha RP. Fabrication of thick film sensitive RuO2-TiO2 and Ag/AgCl/KCl reference electrodes and their application for pH measurements. Sens Actuators B Chem 2014;204:57-67.
[49] Arshak K, Gill E, Arshak A, Korostynska O. Investigation of tin oxides as sensing layers in conductimetric interdigitated pH sensors. Sens Actuators B Chem 2007;127(1):42-53.
[50] Zhuiykov S. Morphology of Pt-doped nanofabricated RuO2 sensing electrodes and their properties in water quality monitoring sensors. Sens Actuators B Chem 2009;136(1):248-56.
[51] Vilouras A, Christou A, Manjakkal L, Dahiya R. Ultrathin ion-sensitive field-effect transistor chips with bending-induced performance enhancement. ACS Appl Electron Mater 2020;2(8):2601-10.

[52] Yin J, Gao W, Zhang Z, Mai Y, Luan A, Jin H, et al. Batch microfabrication of highly integrated silicon-based electrochemical sensor and performance evaluation via nitrite water contaminant determination. Electrochim Acta 2020;335:135660.

[53] Liao YH, Chou JC. Preparation and characteristics of ruthenium dioxide for pH array sensors with real-time measurement system. Sens Actuators B Chem 2008;128(2):603-12.

[54] Manjakkal L, Djurdjic E, Cvejin K, Kulawik J, Zaraska K, Szwagierczak D. Electrochemical impedance spectroscopic analysis of RuO2 based thick film pH sensors. Electrochim Acta 2015;168:246-55.

[55] Korostynska O, Mason A, Al-Shamma'a AI. Flexible microwave sensors for real-time analysis of water contaminants. J Electromagn Waves Appl 2013;27(16):2075-89.

[56] Gill E, Arshak A, Arshak K, Korostynska O. Response mechanism of novel polyaniline composite conductimetric pH sensors and the effects of polymer binder, surfactant and film thickness on sensor sensitivity. Eur Polym J 2010;46(10):2042-50.

[57] Li Y, Mao Y, Xiao C, Xu X, Li X. Flexible pH sensor based on a conductive PANI membrane for pH monitoring. RSC Adv 2020;10(1):21-8.

[58] Yen YK, Lee KY, Lin CY, Zhang ST, Wang CW, Liu TY. Portable nanohybrid paper-based chemiresistive sensor for free chlorine detection. ACS Omega 2020;5(39):25209-15.

[59] Jeon JY, Kang BC, Ha TJ. Flexible pH sensors based on printed nanocomposites of single-wall carbon nanotubes and Nafion. Appl Surf Sci 2020;514:145956.

[60] Devictor V, Whittaker RJ, Beltrame C. Beyond scarcity: citizen science programmes as useful tools for conservation biogeography. Divers Distrib 2010;16(3):354-62.

[61] Qi H, Liu J, Deng Y, Gao S, Mäder E. Cellulose fibres with carbon nanotube networks for water sensing. J Mater Chem A 2014;2(15):5541-7.

[62] Jalbert K, Kinchy AJ. Sense and influence: environmental monitoring tools and the power of citizen science. J Environ Policy Plan. 2016;18(3):379-97.

[63] Silvertown J. A new dawn for citizen science. Trends Ecol Evol 2009;24(9): 467-71.

[64] Bonney R, Cooper CB, Dickinson J, Kelling S, Phillips T, Rosenberg KV, et al. Citizen science: a developing tool for expanding science knowledge and scientific literacy. BioScience 2009;59(11):977-84.

[65] Brossard D, Lewenstein B, Bonney R. Scientific knowledge and attitude change: The impact of a citizen science project. Int J Sci Educ 2005;27(9):1099-121.

[66] Jollymore A, Haines MJ, Satterfield T, Johnson MS. Citizen science for water quality monitoring: Data implications of citizen perspectives. J Environ Manage 2017;200:456-67.

[67] Flanagin AJ, Metzger MJ. The credibility of volunteered geographic information. GeoJournal 2008;72:137-48.

[68] Riesch H, Potter C, Davies L. Combining citizen science and public engagement: The Open Air Laboratories Programme. J Sci Commun 2013;12(3):A03.

[69] Druschke CG, Seltzer CE. Failures of engagement: Lessons learned from a citizen science pilot study. Appl Environ Educ Commun 2012;11(3-4):178-88.
[70] Fazal-ur-Rehman M. Polluted water borne diseases: Symptoms, causes, treatment and prevention. J Med Chem Sci 2019;2(1):21-6.
[71] Cloete TE, Rose JB, Nel L, Ford T. Microbial waterborne pathogens. London: IWA Publishing, 2004.
[72] VanDerslice J. Drinking water infrastructure and environmental disparities: evidence and methodological considerations. Am J Public Health 2011;101(S1):S109-S14.
[73] Shiber JG. Arsenic in domestic well water and health in central Appalachia, USA. Water Air Soil Pollut 2005;160:327-41.
[74] Oyedepo S, Adeyemi G, Olawole O, Ohijeagbon O, Fagbemi O, Solomon R, et al. A GIS-based method for assessment and mapping of noise pollution in Ota metropolis, Nigeria. MethodsX 2019;6:447-57.
[75] Marjanović M, Grubeša S, Žarko IP, editors. Air and noise pollution monitoring in the city of Zagreb by using mobile crowdsensing. 25th International Conference on Software, Telecommunications and Computer Networks (SoftCOM), IEEE, 2017.
[76] Leao S, Ong KL, Krezel A. 2Loud? Community mapping of exposure to traffic noise with mobile phones. Environ Monit Assess 2014;186:6193-206.
[77] Maisonneuve N, Stevens M, Niessen ME, Steels L, editors. NoiseTube: Measuring and mapping noise pollution with mobile phones. In: Information Technologies in Environmental Engineering: Proceedings of the 4th International ICSC Symposium Thessaloniki, Greece, 2009 May 28-29.
[78] Kanjo E. Noisespy: A real-time mobile phone platform for urban noise monitoring and mapping. Mobile Netw Appl 2010;15:562-74.
[79] Rana RK, Chou CT, Kanhere SS, Bulusu N, Hu W, editors. Ear-phone: an end-to-end participatory urban noise mapping system. Proceedings of the 9th ACM/IEEE International Conference on Information Processing in Sensor Networks, 2010.
[80] D'Hondt E, Stevens M, Jacobs A. Participatory noise mapping works! An evaluation of participatory sensing as an alternative to standard techniques for environmental monitoring. Pervasive Mob Comput 2013;9(5):681-94.
[81] Sexton K, Adgate JL. Looking at environmental justice from an environmental health perspective. J Expo Anal Environ Epidemiol 1999;9(1):3-8.
[82] Standl E, Khunti K, Hansen TB, Schnell O. The global epidemics of diabetes in the 21st century: Current situation and perspectives. Eur J Prev Cardiol 2019;26(2_suppl):7-14.
[83] Association AD. 2. Classification and diagnosis of diabetes. Diabetes Care 2017;40(Suppl 1):S11-24.
[84] Hayes C, Kriska A. Role of physical activity in diabetes management and prevention. J Am Diet Assoc 2008;108(4):S19-23.
[85] DeSalvo D, Buckingham B. Continuous glucose monitoring: current use and future directions. Curr Diabetes Rep 2013;13:657-62.

[86] Jagai JS, Krajewski AK, Shaikh S, Lobdell DT, Sargis RM. Association between environmental quality and diabetes in the USA. J Diabetes Investig 2020;11(2):315-24.
[87] Neel BA, Sargis RM. The paradox of progress: environmental disruption of metabolism and the diabetes epidemic. Diabetes 2011;60(7):1838-48.
[88] Calafat AM, Ye X, Wong LY, Reidy JA, Needham LL. Exposure of the US population to bisphenol A and 4-tertiary-octylphenol: 2003–2004. Environ Health Perspect 2008;116(1):39-44.
[89] Ruiz D, Becerra M, Jagai JS, Ard K, Sargis RM. Disparities in environmental exposures to endocrine-disrupting chemicals and diabetes risk in vulnerable populations. Diabetes Care 2018;41(1):193-205.
[90] DIABETES FFO. National Diabetes Fact Sheet, 2011.
[91] Zoeller RT, Brown TR, Doan LL, Gore AC, Skakkebaek NE, Soto AM, et al. Endocrine-disrupting chemicals and public health protection: A statement of principles from The Endocrine Society. Endocrinology 2012;153(9):4097-110.
[92] Silverstone AE, Rosenbaum PF, Weinstock RS, Bartell SM, Foushee HR, Shelton C, et al. Polychlorinated biphenyl (PCB) exposure and diabetes: Results from the Anniston Community Health Survey. Environ Health Perspect 2012;120(5):727-32.
[93] Leff T, Stemmer P, Tyrrell J, Jog R. Diabetes and exposure to environmental lead (Pb). Toxics 2018;6(3):54.
[94] Hanna-Attisha M, LaChance J, Sadler RC, Champney Schnepp A. Elevated blood lead levels in children associated with the Flint drinking water crisis: A spatial analysis of risk and public health response. Am J Public Health 2016;106(2):283-90.
[95] Fridlyand L, Philipson L. Reactive species and early manifestation of insulin resistance in type 2 diabetes. Diabetes Obes Metab 2006;8(2):136-45.
[96] Lee D-H, Lim J-S, Song K, Boo Y, Jacobs Jr DR. Graded associations of blood lead and urinary cadmium concentrations with oxidative-stress–related markers in the US population: Results from the Third National Health and Nutrition Examination Survey. Environ Health Perspect 2006;114(3):350-4.
[97] Khan AR, Awan FR. Metals in the pathogenesis of type 2 diabetes. J Diabetes Metab Disord 2014;13:1-6.
[98] Georgiou K, Larentzakis AV, Khamis NN, Alsuhaibani GI, Alaska YA, Giallafos EJ. Can wearable devices accurately measure heart rate variability? A systematic review. Folia Med 2018;60(1):7-20.
[99] El-Amrawy F, Nounou MI. Are currently available wearable devices for activity tracking and heart rate monitoring accurate, precise, and medically beneficial? Healthc Inform Res 2015;21(4):315-20.
[100] Kong Y, Chon KH. Heart rate tracking using a wearable photoplethysmographic sensor during treadmill exercise. IEEE Access 2019;7:152421-8.
[101] Etiwy M, Akhrass Z, Gillinov L, Alashi A, Wang R, Blackburn G, et al. Accuracy of wearable heart rate monitors in cardiac rehabilitation. Cardiovasc Diagn Ther 2019;9(3):262.

[102] Alugubelli N, Abuissa H, Roka A. Wearable devices for remote monitoring of heart rate and heart rate variability—What we know and what is coming. Sensors 2022;22(22):8903.
[103] Mc Namara K, Alzubaidi H, Jackson JK. Cardiovascular disease as a leading cause of death: how are pharmacists getting involved? Integr Pharm Res Pract 2019;8:1-11.
[104] Virani SS, Alonso A, Benjamin EJ, Bittencourt MS, Callaway CW, Carson AP, et al. Heart disease and stroke statistics—2020 update: a report from the American Heart Association. Circulation 2020;141(9):e139-596.
[105] Gaziano T, Reddy KS, Paccaud F, Horton S, Chaturvedi V. Cardiovascular disease. In: Jamison DT, Breman JG, Measham AR, Alleyne G, Claeson M, Evans DB et al., eds. Disease control priorities in developing countries, 2nd ed. New York: Oxford University Press, 2006.
[106] Daiber A, Lelieveld J, Steven S, Oelze M, Kröller-Schön S, Sørensen M, et al. The "exposome" concept—how environmental risk factors influence cardiovascular health. Acta Biochim Pol 2019;66(3):269-83.
[107] Cosselman KE, Navas-Acien A, Kaufman JD. Environmental factors in cardiovascular disease. Nat Rev Cardiol 2015;12(11):627-42.
[108] Franklin BA, Brook R, Pope III CA. Air pollution and cardiovascular disease. Curr Probl Cardiol 2015;40(5):207-38.
[109] Münzel T, Hahad O, Daiber A, Landrigan PJ. Soil and water pollution and human health: what should cardiologists worry about? Cardiovasc Res 2023;119(2):440-9.
[110] Lawrence DL, Low SM. The built environment and spatial form. Annu Rev Anthropol 1990;19(1):453-505.
[111] Activity NRCCoP, Transportation, Use L, Board TR, Medicine Io. Does the built environment influence physical activity? Examining the evidence--Special report 282. Washington, DC: Transportation Research Board, 2005.
[112] Ewing R, Schmid T, Killingsworth R, Zlot A, Raudenbush S. Relationship between urban sprawl and physical activity, obesity, and morbidity. Am J Health Promot 2003;18(1):47-57.
[113] Hu PS, Young J. Summary of travel trends: 1995 nationwide personal transportation survey. Washington, DC: Federal Highway Administration, 1999.
[114] Lindström M. Means of transportation to work and overweight and obesity: a population-based study in southern Sweden. Prev Med 2008;46(1):22-8.
[115] Sallis JF, Floyd MF, Rodríguez DA, Saelens BE. Role of built environments in physical activity, obesity, and cardiovascular disease. Circulation 2012;125(5):729-37.
[116] Nieuwenhuijsen MJ. Influence of urban and transport planning and the city environment on cardiovascular disease. Nat Rev Cardiol 2018;15(7):432-8.
[117] Ioannidou I, Sklavos N. On general data protection regulation vulnerabilities and privacy issues, for wearable devices and fitness tracking applications. Cryptography 2021;5(4):29.
[118] Raij A, Ghosh A, Kumar S, Srivastava M, editors. Privacy risks emerging from the adoption of innocuous wearable sensors in the mobile environment.

Proceedings of the SIGCHI Conference on Human Factors in Computing Systems, 2011.
[119] Di Pietro R, Mancini LV. Security and privacy issues of handheld and wearable wireless devices. Commun ACM. 2003;46(9):74-9.
[120] Datta P, Namin AS, Chatterjee M, editors. A survey of privacy concerns in wearable devices. 2018 IEEE International Conference on Big Data (Big Data), 2018.
[121] Moon NW, Baker PM, Goughnour K. Designing wearable technologies for users with disabilities: Accessibility, usability, and connectivity factors. J Rehabil Assist Technol Eng 2019;6:2055668319862137.
[122] Kekade S, Hseieh CH, Islam MM, Atique S, Khalfan AM, Li YC, et al. The usefulness and actual use of wearable devices among the elderly population. Comput Methods Programs Biomed 2018;153:137-59.
[123] Iancu I, Iancu B. Designing mobile technology for elderly. A theoretical overview. Technol Forecast Soc Change 2020;155:119977.
[124] Jansen J. Use of the internet in higher-income households. Washington, DC: Pew Research Center, 2010.
[125] Gonzales AL, Ems L, Suri VR. Cell phone disconnection disrupts access to healthcare and health resources: A technology maintenance perspective. New Media Soc 2016;18(8):1422-38.
[126] Tsetsi E, Rains SA. Smartphone Internet access and use: Extending the digital divide and usage gap. Mobile Media Commun 2017;5(3):239-55.
[127] Gandy M, Baker PM, Zeagler C. Imagining futures: A collaborative policy/device design for wearable computing. Futures 2017;87:106-21.
[128] De Zambotti M, Cellini N, Goldstone A, Colrain IM, Baker FC. Wearable sleep technology in clinical and research settings. Med Sci Sports Exerc 2019;51(7):1538.
[129] Abboushi B, Safranek S, Rodriguez-Feo Bermudez E, Pratoomratana S, Chen Y, Poplawski M, et al. A review of the use of wearables in indoor environmental quality studies and an evaluation of data accessibility from a wearable device. Front Built Environ 2022;8:787289.
[130] Carrier B, Barrios B, Jolley BD, Navalta JW. Validity and reliability of physiological data in applied settings measured by wearable technology: A rapid systematic review. Technologies 2020;8(4):70.
[131] Lee J, Kim D, Ryoo HY, Shin BS. Sustainable wearables: Wearable technology for enhancing the quality of human life. Sustainability 2016;8(5):466.
[132] Guida D, Basukoski A, Database P, editors. WEIGHTBIT: An advancement in wearable technology. 2017 IEEE 30th International Symposium on Computer-Based Medical Systems (CBMS), 2017.
[133] Montes J, Tandy R, Young J, Lee S-P, Navalta JW. Step count reliability and validity of five wearable technology devices while walking and jogging in both a free motion setting and on a treadmill. Int J Exerc Sci. 2020;13(7):410.
[134] Blevins B. Teaching digital literacy composing concepts: Focusing on the layers of augmented reality in an era of changing technology. Comput Compos 2018;50:21-38.

[135] Duin AH, Moses J, McGrath M, Tham J. Wearable computing, wearable composing: New dimensions in composition pedagogy. Computers Composition Online 2016. Corpus ID: 226993792.
[136] Ylipulli J, Luusua A, eds. Without libraries what have we? Public libraries as nodes for technological empowerment in the era of smart cities, AI and big data. Proceedings of the 9th International Conference on Communities & Technologies-Transforming Communities, 2019.
[137] Banerjee A, Joshi KP, editors. Link before you share: Managing privacy policies through blockchain. 2017 IEEE International Conference on Big Data (Big Data), 2017.
[138] Baker PM, Gandy M, Zeagler C. Innovation and wearable computing. IEEE Internet Comput 2015;19(5):18-25.

Chapter 3

Occupational determinants of health

Aderonke Adetunji, MS
and Emmanuel Obeng-Gyasi*, PhD, MPH
Department of Built Environment, North Carolina A&T State University, Greensboro, North Carolina, United States of America

Abstract

Occupational determinants of health encompass a broad spectrum of workplace factors that wield considerable influence over an individual's holistic well-being, encompassing physical, mental, and social dimensions. This viewpoint aims to provide an expansive and nuanced examination, evaluation, and definition of these determinants, elucidating the intricate interplay between one's occupation and their health. Extensive research, including a meticulous review of qualitative and quantitative studies conducted between 2000 and 2023, has been undertaken to delineate occupational hazards prevalent across diverse professions. The findings underscore the pivotal roles played by biological and chemical hazards, alongside the intricate web of occupational and socioeconomic factors, in shaping the health landscape of workers. This comprehensive analysis not only highlights the varied dimensions of occupational health but also sheds light on the multifaceted nature of hazards, emphasizing their significant impact on the well-being of individuals within the workforce.

---

* *Correspondence:* Associate professor Emmanuel Obeng-Gyasi, PhD, MPH, Department of Built Environment, North Carolina A&T State University, Greensboro, NC 27411, United States of America. Email: eobenggyasi@ncat.edu

In: Public Health: Understanding the Impact of Environmental Pollutants
Editors: Emmanuel Obeng-Gyasi and Joav Merrick
ISBN: 979-8-89530-579-9
© 2025 Nova Science Publishers, Inc.

Introduction

Occupational determinants of health encompass a spectrum of factors and circumstances found in the workplace that wield substantial influence over an individual's overall health and wellness. These determinants can exert favorable and unfavorable impacts on a person's physical, mental, and social well-being (1). Based on an analysis to estimate the number of United States workers that are frequently exposed to infectious and disease-causing agents in the workplace, the result from the survey showed that as of 2018, of 144.7 million people employed in the United States, approximately 10% (14,425,070) and 18.4% (26,669,810) of workers were exposed to disease or infection at least once per week and once per month respectively (2). It was also noted that the majority of the exposed workers are employed in healthcare sectors and others, including protective service occupations, office and administrative support occupations, education occupations, community and social services occupations, and construction and social services occupations (2). It is important to explore comprehensively how workers are exposed to infectious and disease-causing agents in the workplace and the factors responsible for this.

Occupational hazards negatively impact workers' health; they are classified as physical, biological, chemical, ergonomic, mechanical, and psychosocial hazards (3). Other factors that impact workers' health include physical work environment, organizational, socioeconomic, occupational disparities, occupational health promotion and occupational health protection can have both favorable and unfavorable impact on workers' health (4).

Research has shown diseases and health complications associated with occupations due to exposure to the above-stated hazards at their workplace. Some of the health complications include chemical burns, skin disorders, respiratory problems, anxiety and depression, organ damage, and cancers in some extreme cases of exposure to toxic chemicals (5-7). A research study aimed at examining the impact of physical hazard exposure on the health of forestry vehicle operators engaged in wood logging operations found that 27% of the workers had been diagnosed with a range of health conditions. These conditions included osteo-musculoskeletal disorders, dermatological issues, respiratory problems, and cardiovascular diseases. Among these health issues, osteo-musculoskeletal disorders were the most prevalent. These health problems were attributed to the workers' exposure to workplace hazards, including noise, whole-body vibration, and various environmental elements (8). In another study, occupational hearing impairment was detected among twenty-two million workers, encompassing both men and women aged between 18 and 65. These individuals had been exposed to unsafe noise levels within various industries across the United States (9).

This paper aims to embark on a comprehensive exploration, assessment, and definition of the overarching occupational determinants of health. In doing so, we endeavor to dissect and illuminate the multifaceted aspects that shape an individual's health within the context of their occupation.

To achieve this objective, we will extensively review existing literature, drawing upon various disciplines such as public health, occupational science, sociology, psychology, and epidemiology. This interdisciplinary approach will enable us to identify and comprehensively analyze the diverse factors that influence health outcomes in the workplace.

Our investigation will encompass an exhaustive examination of the physical, psychosocial, and environmental factors that individuals encounter while engaged in their occupations. We will delve into the impact of workplace hazards, ergonomic considerations, and occupational exposures on health. Simultaneously, we will explore the interplay of psychosocial stressors, job satisfaction, work-life balance, and mental well-being in shaping an individual's overall health status. Furthermore, we will scrutinize the role of workplace policies, organizational culture, and access to healthcare resources in this complex equation.

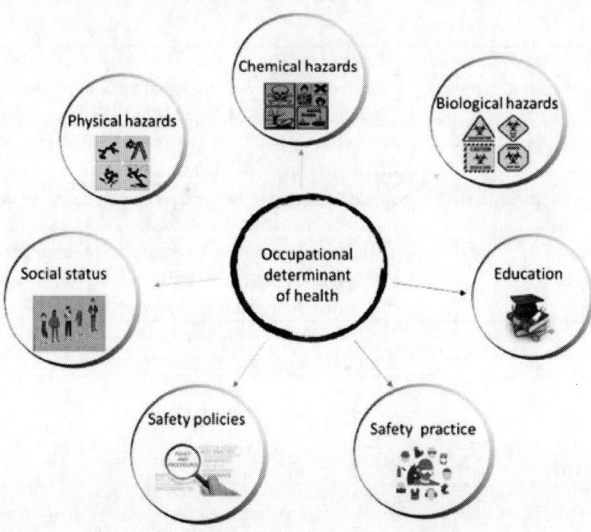

Figure 1. Occupational determinant of health.

By elucidating these multifaceted determinants, we aim to provide a comprehensive framework that not only identifies the factors at play but also defines their collective influence on an individual's health. Figure 1 shows the summary of occupational determinant of health.

Our investigation

In this viewpoint, we aimed to undertake a thorough investigation, evaluation, and clarification of the fundamental occupational factors influencing health. We conducted computer-based searches in academic databases including PubMed and ScienceDirect. To optimize search outcomes, we employed diverse combinations of keywords identified in the literature, Medical Subject Heading (MeSH) and general terms associated with various types of workplace hazards and their health implications. Some of these terms such as occupational health, workplace hazards, prevalence of occupational hazards, physical hazards, chemical hazards, biological hazards, musculoskeletal disorder, COVID-19 pandemic, occupational diseases, and socioeconomic status. The table showing the combination of the searched words can be found in Table 1.

Table 1. Searched words combination

Database	Type of search	Search terms
Google Scholar	General terms	Occupational health, chemical hazard, physical hazard, biological hazard, workplace hazard, socioeconomic status, occupational health, prevalence of work hazard, workplace diseases, preventive measures of workplace injuries.
PubMed database	Medical subject headings	Musculoskeletal disorder, physical hazard, occupational hazard, occupational health risks, work injuries, occupational exposure to diseases, diseases preventive measures, workplace risks reduction, workplace chemical exposure, chemical hazards, work accidents.
ScienceDirect	General terms	Occupational determinant of health, work hazard, work injuries, occupational risk assessments.

Study selection

This viewpoint was conducted a thorough search for qualitative and quantitative studies that reported findings on hazards associated with various occupations spanning from 2000 to 2023. The inclusivity of our search extended to studies conducted both in the United States and internationally. However, to maintain language consistency, studies not published in English language were excluded. The scope of our inquiry aimed to gather comprehensive insights into occupational hazards across diverse settings and geographic locations. The selected timeframe allowed us to capture a broad spectrum of relevant research conducted over the past two decades.

What we found

When searching through Google Scholar, PubMed and ScienceDirect for articles on occupational determinant of health, 63 articles, 46 articles and 49 articles were found from each database respectfully. Our initial search identified a total of 158 articles and identified five records from websites and organizations. After all the duplicate articles and articles that were not eligible were removed, we were left with 103 articles for screening. During the screening of the articles, 26 articles were excluded against titles and abstracts, 27 articles were excluded because we were unable to obtain the full text for our review and seven were excluded because they were not published in English.

In this viewpoint, a total of 48 studies were used to explore how physical hazards, biological hazards, chemical hazards, socioeconomic factors and occupational health promotion and protection at different workplaces and how they affect the health of the workers. Table 2 shows the summary of occupational hazards, sources, health risks and preventive measures.

Of the 48 articles, 10 studies of occupational determinant of health are summarized in Table 3.

Table 2. Occupational health hazards, sources, health risks and preventive measures

Occupational hazards	Sources	Health risks	Preventive measure
Physical hazard	<ul><li>Machinery and Equipment</li><li>Electrical Sources</li><li>Noise and Vibration</li><li>Falling Objects</li><li>Confined Spaces</li><li>Extreme temperatures</li><li>Radiation Sources</li><li>Wet floors</li></ul>	<ul><li>Bruises</li><li>Electric shock</li><li>Burns</li><li>Acute radiation syndrome</li><li>Hearing loss</li><li>Stress and fatigue</li><li>Musculoskeletal disorders</li></ul>	<ul><li>Use of personal protective equipment</li><li>Training on handling Proper of tools and equipment.</li><li>Proper ventilation</li></ul>
Biological hazard	<ul><li>Bloodborne pathogens</li><li>Parasite</li><li>Bacterial</li><li>Virus</li><li>Organic dust and bioaerosols</li></ul>	<ul><li>Infectious diseases such as influenza, tuberculosis, hepatitis, and blood-borne diseases</li><li>Respiratory problem</li><li>Skin Infections</li><li>Gastrointestinal Issues</li></ul>	<ul><li>Use of personal protective equipment</li><li>Vaccination</li><li>Infection Control Practices</li><li>Training</li><li>Routine Cleaning and Disinfection</li><li>Personal Hygiene</li></ul>
Chemical hazard	<ul><li>Toxic chemicals</li><li>Irritants and corrosives</li><li>Carcinogens</li><li>flammable and combustible chemicals</li><li>Mutagenic substances</li></ul>	<ul><li>Respiratory problems</li><li>Organ damage</li><li>Skin burns</li><li>Anthrax</li><li>Aches</li><li>Ulcers in the hand and nose</li><li>Irritation of windpipes</li><li>Cancer</li><li>Genetic mutations</li></ul>	<ul><li>Use of personal protective equipment</li><li>Training and Education</li><li>Proper labeling of chemicals</li><li>Spill Response Kits</li><li>Regular Inspections</li><li>Proper Storage of chemicals</li></ul>

Occupational hazards	Sources	Health risks	Preventive measure
Organizational factors	<ul><li>Workload and Work Pressure</li><li>Job Insecurity</li><li>Workplace Violence and Bullying</li><li>Inadequate Training and Development</li><li>Discrimination and Harassment</li><li>Poor Social Support</li></ul>	<ul><li>Stress</li><li>Anxiety</li><li>Depression</li><li>Hypertension</li><li>Psychological Disorders</li><li>Decreased Productivity</li><li>Increased Risk of Accidents</li></ul>	<ul><li>Leadership and Management Training</li><li>Employee Involvement</li><li>Workload Management</li><li>Support Programs</li><li>Promote a Positive Work Environment</li></ul>

Table 3. Summary of studies for occupational determinants of health

Author	Date	Sample size	Study Design	Findings
Alexopoulos, E. C., Stathi, I. C., & Charizani, F.	2004	430 dentists	A questionnaire survey was carried out among dentists on the respondent's job history, individual characteristics, physical and psychosocial risk factors at work, general health status, and the occurrence of musculoskeletal complaints.	62%, 30%, 16%, and 32% of the dentists reported at least one musculoskeletal complaint, chronic complaints, had spells of absence and, sought medical care respectively.
Baer, R., Turnberg, W., Yu, D., & Wöhrle, R.	2010	1	A veterinarian specializing in small animals in Washington State handled a seemingly healthy pet rat approximately 10 days before falling ill. During the examination, the rat, which appeared free of fleas, urinated on the veterinarian's hands, who was not wearing gloves. Despite washing his hands after the examination, the veterinarian had abrasions from gardening.	The small animal veterinarian developed leptospirosis after occupational exposure. The risk of the infection could have been minimized if he had practiced the recommended infection control procedures
Baker, M. G., Peckham, T. K., & Seixas, N. S.	2020	144.7 million people employed in the United States	The number of United States workers frequently exposed to infection and disease was estimated in the workplace. National employment data by Standard Occupational Classification maintained by the Bureau of Labor Statistics (BLS) was merged with a BLS O*NET survey measure	As of 2018, approximately 10% (14,425,070) and 18.4% (26,669,810) of workers in the United States are exposed to disease or infection at least once per week and once per month respectively
Gibb, H. J., Lees, P. S., Pinsky, P. F., & Rooney, B. C.	2000	2,357 workers first employed between 1950 and 1974	The risk of lung cancer was assed among workers at a chromate production plant. Cumulative trivalent chromium exposure for each individual in the study cohort was estimated.	Cumulative hexavalent chromium exposure showed a strong dose–response relationship for lung cancer.

Author	Date	Sample size	Study Design	Findings
Girard, S. A., Picard, M., Davis, A. C., Simard, M., Larocque, R., Leroux, T., & Turcotte, F.	2009	52,982 male workers between the ages of 16 and 64 years	A retrospective study was conducted on male workers with long-standing exposures to occupational noise over a 5-year period, using "hearing status" and "noise exposure" from the registry held by the Quebec National Institute of Public Health. Information on work-related accidents was obtained from the Quebec Workers' Compensation Board. Hearing threshold level measurements and noise exposures were regressed on the numbers of accidents after adjusting for age.	Exposure to extremely noisy environments (Leq8h (equivalent noise level for 8 h exposure) ≥ 90 dBA) is associated with a higher relative risk of hearing impairment.
Hu, R., Huang, X., Huang, J., Li, Y., Zhang, C., Yin, Y., ... & Cui, F.	2015	246 farmers	Medical doctors conducted two sets of health investigations on the farmers, involving blood tests and neurological examinations, both before and after the crop season. Face-to-face interview was also used to collect data on pesticide use.	Long-term exposure to pesticides was linked to heightened abnormalities in nerve conductions, particularly in sensory nerves. Short-term health effects included alterations in complete blood count, hepatic and renal functions, and nerve conduction velocities and amplitudes.
Meyer, A., Sandler, D. P., Beane Freeman, L. E., Hofmann, J. N., & Parks, C. G.	2017	52,394 private pesticide applicators	Participants provided questionnaire data on the duration, frequency and use of different pesticides. Association of rheumatoid arthritis was evaluated with the use of 46 pesticides.	Incident rheumatoid arthritis was associated with ever use of fonofos, carbaryl and chlorimuron ethyl.

Table 3. (Continued)

Author	Date	Sample size	Study Design	Findings
Oakman, J., Ketels, M., & Clays, E.	2021	331 participants within the service and manufacturing sector in the Flemish Employees' Physical Activity	Data from participants within the service and manufacturing sector in the Flemish Employees' Physical Activity (FEPA) study were collected using objective measures of occupational physical activity and subjective measures of physical and psychosocial work environment. A modified Nordic questionnaire was used to collect data on low back pain (LBP) and neck and shoulder pain (NSP).	Objective measures showed no correlation with LBP or NSP, whereas self-reported measures revealed potential workplace hazards. LBP, NSP and the composite measure of LBP/NSP simultaneously was reported by 25%, 30% and 17% of the participants respectively.
Parks, C. G., Walitt, B. T., Pettinger, M., Chen, J. C., De Roos, A. J., Hunt, J., ... & Howard, B. V.	2011	76,861 postmenopausal women, ages 50–79 years	Incident cases were identified based on self-report and use of disease-modifying antirheumatic drugs at year 3 of follow up. Self-reported residential or workpace insecticide use (personally mixing/applying by self and application by others) in relation to rheumatoid arthritis/ systemic lupus erythematosus (RA/SLE) risk, overall and in relation to farm history was examined.	Personal use of insecticides, long-term insecticide application by others and frequent application by others among women with a farm history were associated with increased RA/SLE risk.
Pettersson, H., Olsson, D., & Järvholm, B.	2020	194,501 workers in the Swedish construction industry	Participants participated in health examinations between 1971 and 1993. The workers answered a questionnaire regarding their working conditions and their health status including height, weight, tobacco use, and blood pressure. Noise exposure data was derived from a survey of working conditions conducted by industrial hygienists in the mid-1970s. Workers were divided into three primary regions in Sweden based on varying temperatures.	Moderate and high noise exposure was associated with increased risk of myocardial infarction and stroke mortality. Living and working in the coldest region was associated with increased risk for myocardial infarction but not stroke mortality.

Discussion

In this chapter we aim to explore the physical, psychosocial, and environmental hazards individuals are exposed to during their engagement in various occupations. Occupational determinants of health encompass a variety of factors inherent in the work environment and employment conditions, exerting a substantial impact on an individual's overall well-being and health outcomes. These determinants include a diverse set of elements associated with one's occupation, workplace, and employment circumstances.

Occupational determinants are closely linked to the broader standardized social determinants of health framework, providing a comprehensive understanding of health disparities and outcomes. One's occupational nature significantly shapes socioeconomic status, a pivotal element of social determinants of health, covering aspects such as income, education, and social standing. The critical determinants within the work environment, encompassing exposure to hazards and job security, emerge as essential factors in the occupational realm that intersect with social determinants of health. The hazards individuals are exposed to at different workplaces are discussed below.

Physical hazards

Physical hazards in the workplace pose risks and dangers to employees due to their physical properties or characteristics, potentially resulting in injuries, health issues, or even death. Despite the serious consequences associated with physical hazards, they are sometimes considered to be of lesser concern when compared to chemical hazards (3). Physical hazards in occupational settings can occur in various forms and circumstances, which can vary depending on the specific workplace environment. Some of these forms include mechanical, electrical, thermal, radiation, noise, and vibration hazards (3). Mechanical hazards involve using equipment and machinery containing moving components capable of shearing, cutting, or crushing, potentially causing harm to individuals operating them. These hazards can lead to a range of injuries, including bruises, cuts, puncture wounds, fractures, head and eye injuries, as well as back and spinal injuries, among others (10). Physical hazards related to electricity can be caused by faulty electrical equipment, exposed wire or bad or damaged wiring system causing electric shock, burns, electrocution, internal injuries, or death (11). Thermal and radiation hazards are caused by extreme cold or hot temperatures and ionizing or non-ionizing radiation exposure (12). Thermal hazards can lead to health issues such as heat exhaustion, heat stroke, frostbite, hypothermia, and burns, whereas radiation hazards can cause conditions in cancer, acute radiation syndrome, radiation burns, cataracts and radiation sickness (12). Noise hazard occurs as a result of exposure to excessive noise in a work environment over a prolonged period of time, it could be from industrial machinery, construction activities, power tools, or firearms among others (13). Exposure to prolonged noise at workplace could cause stress and fatigue, sleep disturbance, hearing loss, cardiovascular effect such as high blood pressure and heart disease etc. (13). Vibration hazard occurs due to workers' exposure to continuous vibration over a long period of time. The vibration can be from different sources such as equipment, vehicles, tools or machinery (14). Vibration can occur as whole-body vibration, where the entire body is in contact with the vibration surface like vehicle seat usually in construction, transportation and agriculture or hand-arm vibration, where the vibration only affects the arm when using vibrating hand tools (14). The health effects associated with whole-body and hand-arm vibration are musculoskeletal disorders, circulatory problems, neurological problems, Raynaud's phenomenon, neurological problems, fatigue and reduced work performance (8, 14). Extensive research has revealed the consequences of workers' exposure to physical hazards in various occupational settings and the resulting adverse effects on their well-being.

In a study to explore the role of occupational physical activity, physical demand, and psychosocial work-related factors on low back pain and neck-shoulder pain amongst workers with physically demanding professions, data was collected from 331 participants comprising of 142 males and 189 females between the age of 20 and 65 within the service and manufacturing sector in the Flemish Employees' Physical Activity using a modified Nordic questionnaire on low back pain and neck-shoulder pain. Using objective measures to evaluate physical activity, two accelerometers were positioned on the middle of the back and right thigh and worn continuously for 3-4 days. Using subjective measures, participants were requested to maintain a diary documenting their daily activities. Psychosocial work factors, such as job demands, job control, and social support, were assessed using constructs from job content questionnaire. Musculoskeletal pain information concerning the lower back and neck-shoulder regions was collected through a modified version of the Standardized Nordic questionnaire, which is used to assess musculoskeletal symptoms. This study showed that about 25% of the participants reported low back pain for more than 30 days during the last year, 30% reported neck-shoulder pain and 17% reported a combination of low back and neck-shoulder pain. Objective measures showed that 37% of workers with physically demanding jobs were standing most of the time, followed by 30.4% sitting and 14.5% performing moderate-to-vigorous physical activity. No correlation was found between objective measures and the occurrence of low back and neck-shoulder pain. However, self-reported measures offered valuable insights into potential workplace hazards, including physical demands and job control, which can inform the development of future strategies to prevent the onset of low back pain and neck-shoulder pain (15).

In another study, a retrospective study of 52,982 male workers between the ages of 16 and 64 years who had experienced prolonged exposure to occupational noise over a period of 5 years was done using hearing status and noise exposure from the registry held by the Quebec National Institute of Public Health to investigate any relationship between noise exposure levels in the workplace, degree of hearing loss, and the relative risk of accident. After accounting for age, a regression analysis was conducted to examine the relationship between hearing threshold level measurements, noise exposures, and the incidence of accidents. From this study, it was shown that the proportion of workers with mild-to-severe hearing loss is higher among the workers exposed to the higher noise level of ≥90 dBA, indicating that the likelihood of high-frequency hearing impairment rises with increasing levels of noise exposure, in line with what is anticipated in cases of noise-induced hearing loss. Additionally, from this study it was indicated that occupational noise exposure has a detrimental impact on workplace safety. It substantially elevates the likelihood of both single and multiple accidents, adding to the well-documented consequences of noise exposure on hearing (16).

Another study was conducted to examine the possible association between occupational exposure to noise, working and living in cold conditions, and the risk of mortality in myocardial infarction and stroke among workers in the Swedish construction industry who participated in health examinations between 1971 and 1993. As method, 194,501 workers answered a questionnaire regarding their working conditions and their health status. A job exposure matrix was created to categorize 21 different work groups in a cohort based on their noise exposure levels. The noise exposure data was derived from a survey of working conditions conducted by industrial hygienists in the mid-1970s. Noise categories were assigned to each working group on a scale of 1 to 5, with levels 1 to 3 representing acceptable noise exposure (45-75 dB(A), level 4 indicating exposure in the range of 76-85 dB(A), and level 5 signifying exposure above 85 dB(A). For analysis purposes, these noise categories were grouped into low (≤75 dB(A)), moderate (76-85 dB(A)), and high (>85 dB(A)) levels. The study highlights a correlation between working in environments with hazardous noise levels and residing and working in cold conditions, leading to an elevated risk of mortality in cases of myocardial infarction evidenced by increased myocardial infarction and stroke mortality with both moderate (76–85 dB) and high noise exposure (> 85 dB). There was a significant increase in myocardial infarction in the coldest region. Noise exposure and climate region interacted to increase the risk of myocardial infarction, with the highest risks observed in individuals exposed to high noise levels while living and working in cold climates. The greatest relative risk of myocardial infarction occurred in the coldest region among those with the highest noise exposure however, this interaction did not affect stroke mortality (17).

The relations between physical, psychosocial and individual characteristics and different endpoints of prevalence of musculoskeletal disorder complaints of low back, neck, shoulders and hand or wrist was investigated in dentists. Musculoskeletal disorders encompass various medical conditions affecting the musculoskeletal system, including both soft tissues (muscles, tendons, ligaments) and hard tissues (bones). These disorders can lead to issues such as pain, inflammation, and reduced mobility. Soft tissue problems may involve inflammation or tears, while hard tissue conditions include fractures, arthritis, or osteoporosis. Overall, musculoskeletal disorders emphasize the interconnectedness of both soft and hard body tissues in maintaining musculoskeletal health. A survey involving 430 dentists in Thessaloniki, Greece, with an 88% response rate, collected data on physical and psychosocial workload, need for recovery, perceived general health, and musculoskeletal complaints in the past year. Logistic regression analysis was used to estimate odds ratios for various risk factors related to these complaints, including chronic issues lasting at least one month, complaints leading to sickness absence, and the seeking of medical care. As result, the physical load among the dentists seems to put them at risk for occurrence of musculoskeletal disorders with the result from the questionnaire showing that from the total of 430 participants, 62% of all subjects reported at least one musculoskeletal complaint, 35% reported at least two musculoskeletal complaints, 15% reported at least three musculoskeletal complaints and 6% reported spells of all four complaints in the past 12 months. Subjects with back pain more often reported neck pain (41%) and hand/wrist pain (38%) than those without back pain (13% and 16%, respectively). Neck and hand/wrist pain was strongly associated since 50% of subjects with neck pain also experienced hand/wrist pain in the past 12 months. Dentists' physical workload appears to increase their risk of musculoskeletal disorders. Severe and multiple complaints are linked to their general health perception, while high perceived exertion and social factors are connected to sickness absence. Chronic symptoms play a role in seeking medical care. Preventing hand/wrist complaints may benefit from ergonomic interventions. When studying the impact of work-related risk factors on musculoskeletal health, it's important to consider psychosocial and personal characteristics (18).

Biological hazards

Biological hazards are health risks associated with exposure to biological agents or pathogens, substances or processes such as bacteria, viruses, fungi, toxins and biological materials in the workplace that can cause acute or chronic health conditions. The presence of biological hazards in the workplace represents a substantial risk to the well-being and safety of employees, raising valid concerns about the potential transmission of these dangers to fellow workers (19). For instance, individuals in healthcare, laboratory and research roles, as well as those in the food industry, may encounter elevated exposure risks of biological hazards (20). Other occupations and industries affected by biological hazards include agriculture and farming, construction, veterinarians and animal handlers, and wastewater and sewage treatment personnel (19). Healthcare workers are faced with potential exposure to bloodborne pathogens such as HIV, hepatitis B, and hepatitis C when they come into contact with contaminated bodily fluids. In laboratory environments, there is inherent proximity to biological agents (20, 21).

Scientists and laboratory staff frequently handle microorganisms, cultures, and samples that may harbor infectious diseases, resulting in the potential risk of biological hazards. Biological hazards within the food industry are linked to product contamination during processing, if not effectively controlled, pathogens such as Escherichia coli and salmonella can give rise to foodborne illnesses, causing significant health concerns (22). In the agricultural and waste management sectors, employees are primarily subjected to organic dust and bioaerosols. Bioaerosols are defined as suspended airborne particles consisting of biological matter, which may include bacterial cells, cellular remnants such as endotoxins, fungal spores, fungal hyphae, viruses, and the metabolic by-products of microorganisms. Additionally, pollen grains and other forms of biological materials can also become airborne as bioaerosols (23).

Occupational biological hazards can be transmitted to workers through various means. These include direct contact with contaminated surfaces, equipment, or co-workers who may carry infectious agents. Additionally, there is the risk of airborne transmission of respiratory pathogens, such as tuberculosis or COVID-19, through the inhalation of infectious droplets. Inadequate ventilation and close proximity to infected individuals can exacerbate this risk (20, 21). Fomite transmission involves inanimate objects carrying biological hazards and can occur through shared equipment, doorknobs, or breakroom utensils. Foodborne transmission is a concern when biological hazards contaminate food products or when proper food hygiene practices are not followed (21). Furthermore, bloodborne pathogens can be transmitted through accidental needlestick injuries or contact with contaminated blood. Certain procedures, like suctioning, can lead to the generation of respiratory droplets containing infectious agents, facilitating droplet spread (20). (24) reported a female patient, aged 40, was diagnosed with tuberculosis in the middle ear on the right side. She had been employed as a nurse at the Department of Pulmonology, Clinical Hospital Rijeka in Rijeka, Croatia, for a duration of 17 years. The infection was attributed to Mycobacterium tuberculosis, acquired during her assistance in bronchoscopy, and was officially recognized as an occupational disease. An outbreak of pertussis was also documented, with transmission occurring among healthcare workers in an oncology department of a hospital, potentially originating from a patient identified as the probable source (25).

In Washington State, a veterinarian specializing in small animals contracted leptospirosis following an incident at work. Roughly 10 days before the onset of the illness, he handled a seemingly healthy pet rat to check for fleas, which urinated on his ungloved hands. Despite washing his hands after the examination, the veterinarian had abrasions on his hands from gardening (26). Ensuring the prevention of biological hazards in the workplace is essential for safeguarding the health and well-being of employees, thereby lowering the chances of illness and potential long-term health impacts.

In the workplace, it is imperative to ensure the safeguarding of employees from biological hazards. Protective measures should be implemented to preclude the possibility of exposure to biological agents and hazards. Where complete prevention may not be feasible, steps should be taken to minimize the risk of exposure to an acceptable level. Control measures encompass systems and actions to minimize exposure risks to biological agents and hazards including engineering controls, management controls and personal protective equipment (19, 27). Engineering controls involves the use of mechanical or physical systems to mitigate the risk of exposure to occupational biological hazards. engineering controls for biological hazards include ventilation systems, biological safety cabinets, airborne infection isolation room, decontamination, handwashing and sterilization equipment, and physical barriers such as shields and screens (19). Management controls aimed at mitigating biological hazards in the workplace encompass administrative and organizational strategies with the primary goal of diminishing risks and safeguarding employee safety. These strategies are intended to formulate clear policies, protocols, and guidelines to ensure the effective management of biological hazards. Examples of management controls include risk assessment, written policies and procedures, training, standard operating procedures, emergency response plan, access control to areas where biological hazards are present, and supervision (19).

Personal protective equipment consists of a range of specialized gear and wear that workers utilize to protect themselves from potential hazards. Personal protective equipment include mask, gowns, eye protection, appropriate footwear, hearing protector and gloves (27). Collectively, these measures serve to reduce the likelihood of employees being exposed to biological hazards in the workplace and contribute to establishing a safer environment for them.

The onset of the COVID-19 pandemic, resulting from infection with the novel coronavirus SARS-CoV-2, marked by various symptoms including fever, cough, breathing issues, and fatigue, has spurred a global prioritization of managing biological risks in occupational environments (28, 29). This underscored the urgent requirement for the development of comprehensive standards and guidelines to effectively tackle these challenges. Considering this situation, companies had to consider their respective national governments' health contingency plans as well as the recommendations of the World Health Organization (WHO) and the International Labor Organization (ILO) (29, 30). This approach was crucial for achieving a necessary balance between reopening operations and the imperative of maintaining low infection rates. The achievement of this balance heavily depended on workers' awareness and the implementation of measures to safeguard their health. Occupational safety and health (OSH) practitioners hold a crucial position in strategizing for the maintenance of secure work environments and in offering guidance and technical support to companies, workers, and their representatives on matters concerning the intricate connection between health and work. Their efforts are primarily concentrated in two key domains, including the recognition and evaluation of occupational hazards (stemming from work-related activities) and the evaluation of individuals' health conditions in the workplace (28).

The emergence of the coronavirus era highlighted the necessity of safeguarding at-risk workers from occupational hazards, particularly those posed by biological factors. Assessing biological risks entails gathering personal data from employees, understanding their health vulnerabilities, and considering their biological condition to accurately evaluate evolving risks (28). This information is vital for devising essential preventive measures and implementing protective protocols. These events have raised awareness and led to changes in workplace safety practices to minimize the risk of virus transmission and protect employees at different levels. Some of these changes include the adoption of remote work arrangements to reduce the number of employees physically present at workplaces, maintaining of a safe distance between employees, wearing of masks to prevent the spread of respiratory droplets, frequent handwashing, sanitizing and good personal hygiene practices, screening and temperature checks to identify potential case, increased cleaning and disinfection, improved ventilation, and workplace safety training (31, 32).

Chemical hazards

Chemical hazards in the workplace are a prevalent worry across multiple industries, presenting dangers to employees' well-being and the work environment's overall stability. These hazards include contact with various chemical compounds, such as harmful substances, combustible elements, corrosive materials, etc. Over 30 million employees within the United States are subject to unsafe chemicals in their workplace (33). The 2021 data addendum reveals that in 2019, exposure to specific chemicals resulted in the loss of approximately two million lives and 53 million disability-adjusted life-years. Nearly 50% of the deaths linked to chemical exposures that year were primarily caused by lead exposure, leading to cardiovascular diseases (34). Employees can be exposed to chemicals at the workplace through inhalation, eye contact, skin contact, ingestion, and injection (35). Exposure to chemicals at work can have several effects on health, ranging from skin burns, anthrax, aches, ulcers in the hand and nose, irritation of windpipes, and cancer (36).

Hazardous workplace chemicals vary based on the work environment. These pose significant health risks, highlighting the need to understand the different types and potential consequences. These chemical hazards are categorized as toxic, corrosive, irritant, carcinogenic, flammable, and mutagenic (36). Toxic chemicals are commonly present in chemical manufacturing, agriculture, and mining industries, where substances like solvents and pesticides are utilized (37,38). Exposure to these toxins can lead to both acute and chronic health issues, such as respiratory problems, organ damage, and even cancer. Irritants and corrosives, on the other hand, encompass chemicals like strong acids, cleaning agents, and alkalis, which find application in industries like manufacturing, cleaning, and metalworking (36). Carcinogens are used in many industries like healthcare, construction, and laboratories. Some of these carcinogens include asbestos, formaldehyde, and certain solvents. Prolonged exposure to carcinogenic substances poses a serious threat to workers' health as it can lead to the development of cancer (39). In industries such as chemical plants, oil refineries, and automotive repair shops, the use of flammable and combustible chemicals like gasoline, aerosols, and propane increases the risk of exposure, potentially resulting in burns, asphyxiation, or even fatalities (40).

Mutagenic substances encountered in workplaces can cause DNA changes and genetic mutations in exposed individuals, significantly elevating the risk of enduring health issues, including a variety of cancers. Exposure to these mutagenic substances in the workplace can have long-lasting and profound health consequences, with the substances encompassing a wide array of chemicals, ranging from specific solvents and heavy metals to pharmaceuticals and even ionizing radiation, such as X-rays and gamma rays (40,41).

Several studies have been conducted to determine the effect of chemical exposure on individuals in the workplace. In research conducted by Herman Gibb and fellow researchers, the objective was to assess the lung cancer risk associated with exposure to both trivalent and hexavalent chromium among individuals employed in chromium production facilities. They examined a cohort comprising 2,357 workers who were initially hired between 1950 and 1974 at a chromate production plant, and the vital status of these workers was tracked until December 31, 1992. From examining the cohort, a progressive relationship between cumulative hexavalent exposure and the incidence of lung cancer was indicated (39). According to Van Rooy et al. (42), the development of bronchiolitis obliterans syndrome among chemical process operators was attributed to their exposure to diacetyl during its manufacturing for food flavorings (42). Armando Meyer and his team conducted a study examining the correlation between the risk of rheumatoid arthritis and the utilization of pesticides among male pesticide applicators enrolled between 1993 and 1997. The study found that heightened occurrences of rheumatoid arthritis were linked to exposure to various pesticides, including fonofos, carbaryl, and imuran ethyl (38). In a similar study, Parks et al. (43) observed an elevated risk of rheumatoid arthritis and the associated condition, systemic lupus erythematosus, in women who self-reported using insecticides during the Women's Health Initiative Observational Study. This risk was more pronounced in women with a farming background. In a sample of the US population as part of the National Health and Nutrition Examination Survey, increased serum levels of organochlorine insecticides were linked to self-reported cases of arthritis, including rheumatoid arthritis (43).

Long-term pesticide exposure was linked to increased abnormalities in nerve conduction, particularly in sensory nerves. This extended exposure also broadly impacted various health indicators based on blood tests. It resulted in reduced amplitudes of the tibial nerve's compound muscle action potential. Short-term exposure had immediate health effects, including changes in complete blood count, hepatic and renal functions, and alterations in nerve conduction velocities and amplitudes (44).

The exposure to chemical hazards originating from coal combustion emissions and diesel engine exhaust was determined to be correlated with urinary mutagenicity, which in turn was associated with an increased risk and development of cancer at multiple locations in the body (40). Therefore, reducing employees' exposure to chemical hazards within their workplace is crucial. Emerging chemical hazards in various industries arise from new chemical compounds, processes, and evolving risk awareness. They can result from innovative chemicals, processes, or the discovery of previously unrecognized risks in existing substances. It is crucially important to adopt a forward-looking strategy to anticipate potential risks posed by chemicals to the health and safety of workers within an ever-evolving work landscape.

With the constant changes in work, an imminent requirement exists to proactively identify potential hazards that may not yet be known or expected. Early detection and alerts can significantly mitigate the likelihood of severe consequences in terms of negative health impacts and broader socio-economic ramifications. Some of the emerging chemicals include nanomaterials, per- and polyfluoroalkyl substances (PFAS), and metal-organic frameworks (MOFs). In recent years, there has been a growing interest in the use of nanotechnology. Nanotechnology involves manipulating matter at scales below 100 nm, resulting in nanoparticles with high surface area-to-volume ratios that enhance reactivity and affect chemical reaction rates (45). Nanomaterials, owing to their unique and beneficial characteristics encompassing chemical reactivity (due to their small size), ductility, flexibility, optical properties, biocompatibility, tunability, enhanced strength, and improved magnetic attributes, offer versatile applications across an array of industries. These applications span diverse fields, including electronics, medicine, energy, aerospace, food production, textiles, cosmetics, and construction (46). PFAS, or per- and polyfluoroalkyl substances, represent a group of artificially produced chemicals. Typically, they contain a carbon chain with most carbon sites saturated by fluorine atoms, along with at least one functional group, like carboxylic acid, sulfonic acid, or amine.

It is important to note that the carbon backbone may not be exclusively carbon; for instance, ether-type PFAS include oxygen atoms in their structure (47). Due to their high production costs, PFAS are typically employed in scenarios where alternative substances are unable to meet the necessary performance standards, or where PFAS can function effectively in much smaller quantities compared to non-fluorinated chemicals while delivering the same level of performance. For instance, they are utilized in applications that operate across broad temperature ranges and in situations that demand exceptionally stable and non-reactive materials (48). PFAS have gained widespread usage across more than 200 application areas, ranging from industrial-mining operations to food production and fire-fighting foams. The key driving force behind the extensive adoption of PFAS lies in the remarkable properties associated with the carbon-fluorine (C-F) bond, which imparts exceptional chemical and thermal stability and the unique ability to repel oil and water (48). MOFs are ordered crystalline materials characterized by structured networks. These frameworks are composed of single metal ions or clusters linked together by multidentate organic groups (49). Their distinct characteristics, such as their expansive surface area, adjustable porosity, and varied chemical compositions, render them applicable across various fields (49). These fields include gas storage and purification, catalysis, drug delivery, energy storage, electronics, coating and films, photocatalysis, and hydrogen storage (49, 50).

Organizational factors

Organizational factors concerning occupational hazards encompass components within an organization's structure, policies, and practices that either amplify or alleviate the risks and threats encountered by employees in the workplace. These factors wield substantial influence over the health and safety of workers. Organizational factors in the workplace wield considerable influence on employee well-being across various dimensions. From a physical standpoint, conditions such as subpar ergonomics, inadequate safety measures, and excessive workloads can contribute to injuries and musculoskeletal disorders (51).

On a mental level, challenges such as overwhelming job demands, job insecurity, and insufficient social support may precipitate stress, anxiety, and depression (52). Psychosocially, the existence of a negative organizational culture, instances of workplace bullying, and discriminatory practices can collectively foster a hostile environment, further impacting mental health (53). The emergence of these health complications emphasizes the intricate interplay among physical, mental, and psychosocial factors within the workplace. Ultimately, it is imperative to address these organizational factors to cultivate a healthier work environment and enhance the overall well-being of employees.

Socioeconomic factors

Socioeconomic factors in the workplace encompass the social and economic conditions shaping the work environment, employment opportunities, and overall well-being of individuals. These factors, including social status, economic position, and resource access, impact various aspects of work life. Considerations such as income level, education, job security, and social support networks play a major role, significantly influencing the type of work individuals engage in and their occupational health outcomes (54).

These socioeconomic factors exert a profound impact on health determinants within the occupational context, influencing access to resources and opportunities. In the sphere of occupational health, these factors shape the nature of work, the quality of employment conditions, and overall well-being (55). Individuals of higher socioeconomic status often find themselves in less hazardous occupations with superior working conditions, while those with lower socioeconomic status may face precarious employment arrangements and increased exposure to occupational risks. This socioeconomic gradient extends to healthcare access, with higher-status individuals benefiting from better preventive care and potentially improved health outcomes (55).

Recognizing and addressing these socioeconomic factors is crucial for fostering health equity and implementing interventions to enhance the overall well-being of the workforce. By acknowledging disparities rooted in socioeconomic factors, initiatives can be tailored to bridge gaps and promote a more inclusive and health-conscious work environment, integral for cultivating a workplace prioritizing the health and prosperity of all its members.

Occupational health promotion and protection

Occupational health promotion involves taking proactive steps in the workplace to improve the overall well-being of employees. This includes creating a positive work environment, promoting healthy behaviors, and preventing health issues before they occur (56). When addressing occupational hazards, health promotion activities may consist of implementing wellness programs, initiatives to manage stress, interventions to improve ergonomics, and educational campaigns to inform employees about potential workplace risks. The objective is to empower workers to make healthier choices and establish a work environment that fosters both their physical and mental health (56).

Occupational health protection on the other hand entails implementing preventive measures and safeguards to reduce or eliminate risks associated with workplace hazards (57). This involves following safety protocols, using personal protective equipment (PPE), adhering to occupational health and safety standards, and identifying and controlling potential hazards. The goal of occupational health protection is to guarantee the physical safety of workers, prevent accidents and injuries, and shield against the harmful effects of occupational exposures. It encompasses the establishment of a secure and hazard-free work environment through activities such as risk assessment, hazard control, and the enforcement of safety regulations (57).

Integrating occupational health determinants with standardized social determinants of health

The review extensively discusses the myriad occupational hazards – physical, biological, chemical, and organizational – and their profound impact on workers' health. These hazards, ranging from exposure to harmful substances to psychosocial stressors, significantly affect the health and well-being of individuals across various occupations.

Comparing these findings with the standard social determinants of health (SDOH), it's evident that occupational determinants of health are intricately intertwined with these broader social factors. For instance, socioeconomic status, a key element of SDOH, is directly influenced by one's occupation, which in turn affects access to resources, healthcare, and overall quality of life. Job security, workplace conditions, and exposure to occupational hazards contribute significantly to health disparities.

However, the CDC's SDOH framework, which includes economic stability, education access and quality, healthcare access and quality, neighborhood and built environment, and social and community context, notably omits specific mention of occupational factors. This exclusion is significant because the nature of one's occupation can profoundly impact overall health, both through direct exposure to hazards and indirectly through socio-economic pathways.

For example, individuals in lower socioeconomic positions often engage in more hazardous jobs due to limited options, leading to increased health risks. This demonstrates a clear intersection between occupational and social determinants of health. Moreover, workplace environments, job security, and conditions significantly influence mental health, stress levels, and overall well-being, further tying occupational factors to broader SDOH.

Conclusion

In conclusion, delving into the occupational determinants of health highlights the complex and multifaceted interconnection between work and well-being. This review's comprehensive exploration of various occupational hazards – from physical to psychosocial and environmental – unequivocally demonstrates their profound impact on individual health outcomes. These findings align with and extend the existing framework of social determinants of health.

The results of this study compellingly justify the inclusion of occupational factors in the standardized list of SDOH. They reveal that occupational determinants, often overlooked, are as influential as other recognized social determinants like economic stability and education access. In many instances, the nature of one's occupation directly influences socio-economic status, access to healthcare, and living conditions, thereby intersecting with, and exacerbating other SDOH.

As workers navigate a dynamic work environment marked by diverse occupations and evolving demands, it becomes increasingly evident that the well-being of the workforce is intrinsically linked to broader social health determinants. This viewpoint contributes to the ongoing discourse on occupational health, urging a re-evaluation of traditional SDOH frameworks to encompass occupational factors. Ultimately, recognizing the role of occupational determinants in public health is not only an ethical imperative but also a strategic investment in enhancing the overall health and productivity of the population.

Acknowledgments

Conceptualization, E.O.-G.; methodology, A.A. and E.O.-G.; formal analysis, A.A.; investigation, A.A. and E.O.-G.; resources, E.O.-G.; data curation, A.A.; writing—original draft preparation, A.A.; writing—review and editing, A.A. and E.O.-G.; supervision, E.O.-G.; project administration, E.O.-G.; funding acquisition, E.O.-G. All authors have read and agreed to the published version of the manuscript. Funding: Research reported in this publication was supported by the National Institute of General Medical Sciences of the National Institutes of Health under Award Number R16GM149473. The content is solely the responsibility of the authors and does not necessarily represent the official views of the National Institutes of Health.

References

[1] Dobson M, Schnall P, Faghri P, Landsbergis P. The Healthy Work Survey: A standardized questionnaire for the assessment of workplace psychosocial hazards and work organization in the United States. J Occup Environ Med 2023;65(5):e330-45.

[2] Baker MG, Peckham TK, Seixas NS. Estimating the burden of United States workers exposed to infection or disease: A key factor in containing risk of COVID-19 infection. PLoS One 2020;15(4):e0232452.

[3] Kumar R, Karthick R, Bhuvaneswari V, Nandhini NJIRJET. Study on occupational health and diseases in oil industry. Int Res J Eng Technol 2017;4(12):954-8.

[4] Blacker A, Dion S, Grossmeier J, Hecht R, Markle E, Meyer L, et al. Social determinants of health—an employer priority. Am J Public Health 2020;34(2):207-15.

[5] Laney AS, Weissman DN. Respiratory diseases caused by coal mine dust. J Occup Environ Med 2014;56(Suppl 10):S18-22.

[6] Dumas O, Varraso R, Boggs KM, Quinot C, Zock JP, Henneberger PK, et al. Association of occupational exposure to disinfectants with incidence of chronic obstructive pulmonary disease among US female nurses. JAMA Network Open 2019;2(10):e1913563-e.

[7] Stamatakis E, Chau JY, Pedisic Z, Bauman A, Macniven R, Coombs N, et al. Are sitting occupations associated with increased all-cause, cancer, and cardiovascular disease mortality risk? A pooled analysis of seven British population cohorts. PLoS One 2013;8(9):e73753.

[8] Iftime MD, Dumitrascu AE, Dumitrascu DI, Ciobanu VDJIJoIE. An investigation on major physical hazard exposures and health effects of forestry vehicle operators performing wood logging processes. Int J Industr Ergonomics 2020;80:103041.

[9] Masterson EA, Tak S, Themann CL, Wall DK, Groenewold MR, Deddens JA, et al. Prevalence of hearing loss in the United States by industry. Am J Ind Med 2013;56(6):670-81.

[10] Gitawangi SV, Ardyanto D. Description of work instructions as part of the mechanical hazard risk control in a construction company. Indonesian J Occupat Saf Health 2022;11(3):367-76.

[11] Rafique R, Sehar S, Afzal M. Health hazards at work place: Application of WHO modal with literature. Saudi J Nurs Health Care 2019;2(12):438-42.

[12] Nakum S, Bhatt M, Ganatra V, Yadav K. Health hazards due to electromagnetic radiation in the workplace. Int J Innovat Res Sci Technol 2015;1(8):138-45.

[13] Gopinath B, Thiagalingam A, Teber E, Mitchell PJPm. Exposure to workplace noise and the risk of cardiovascular disease events and mortality among older adults. Prev Med 2011;53(6):390-4.
[14] Wilder DG, Wasserman DEJP. Occupational vibration exposure. In: Stave GM, Wald PH, eds. Physical and biological hazards of the workplace. New York: Wiley, 2016:53-71.
[15] Oakman J, Ketels M, Clays E. Low back and neck pain: objective and subjective measures of workplace psychosocial and physical hazards. Int Arch Occup Environ Health 2021;94(7):1637-44.
[16] Girard SA, Picard M, Davis AC, Simard M, Larocque R, Leroux T, et al. Multiple work-related accidents: tracing the role of hearing status and noise exposure. Occup Environ Med 2009;66(5):319-24.
[17] Pettersson H, Olsson D, Järvholm BJIAoO, Health E. Occupational exposure to noise and cold environment and the risk of death due to myocardial infarction and stroke. Int Arch Occupat Environ Health 2020;93:571-5.
[18] Alexopoulos EC, Stathi IC, Charizani F. Prevalence of musculoskeletal disorders in dentists. BMC Musculoskelet Disord 2004;5(1):16.
[19] Rim KT, Lim CHJS, work ha. Biologically hazardous agents at work and efforts to protect workers' health: a review of recent reports. Saf Health Work 2014;5(2):43-52.
[20] Walton AL, Rogers B. Workplace hazards faced by nursing assistants in the United States: A focused literature review. Int J Environ Res Public Health 2017;14(5):544.
[21] Chan EYY, Dubois C, Fong AHY, Shaw R, Chatterjee R, Dabral A, et al. Reflection of challenges and opportunities within the COVID-19 pandemic to include biological hazards into DRR planning. Int J Environ Res Public Health 2021;18(4):1614.
[22] Satrio T, Wardhani PJN. Health hazard identification in university research laboratory: A literature review. NeuroQuantology. 2023;21(1):328-35.
[23] Stetzenbach LD. Airborne infectious microorganisms. Encyclopedia Microbiology 2009:175-82.
[24] Lalić H, Kukuljan M, Pavičić MD. A case report of occupational middle ear tuberculosis in a nurse. Arch Industr Hyg Toxicol 2010;61(3):333-7.
[25] Baugh V, McCarthy N. Outbreak of Bordetella pertussis among oncology nurse specialists. Occupat Med 2010;60(5):401-5.
[26] Baer R, Turnberg W, Yu D, Wohrle R. Leptospirosis in a small animal veterinarian: Reminder to follow standardized infection control procedures. Zoonoses Public Health 2010;57(4):281-4.
[27] World Health Organization. Personal protective equipment. Geneva: WHO, 2020.
[28] Carvalhais C, Querido M, Pereira CC, Santos J. Biological risk assessment: A challenge for occupational safety and health practitioners during the COVID-19 (SARS-CoV-2) pandemic. Work 2021;69(1):3-13.
[29] World Health Organization. Rolling updates on coronavirus disease (COVID-19), 2020. URL: https://www.who.int/emergencies/diseases/novel-coronavirus-2019/events-as-they-happen.

[30] World Health Organization. Tripartite validation of the technical guidelines on biological hazards, 2022. URL: https://www.ilo.org/global/topics/safety-and-health-at-work/events-training/events-meetings/WCMS_846243/lang--en/index.htm.

[31] Billock RM, Groenewold MR, Free H, Sweeney MH, Luckhaupt SE. Required and voluntary occupational use of hazard controls for COVID-19 prevention in non–health care workplaces—United States, June 2020. MMWR 2021;70(7):250-3.

[32] Edgar M, Selvaraj SA, Lee KE, Caraballo-Arias Y, Harrell M, Rodriguez-Morales AJ. Healthcare workers, epidemic biological risks-recommendations based on the experience with COVID-19 and Ebolavirus. Infez Med 2022;30(2):168-79.

[33] Subcommittee on Employment, Safety and Training. Hazard communication in the 21st century workplace. Washington, DC: US Government, 2004.

[34] Pan American Health Organization. Chemical safety. Washington, DC: PAHO/WHO, 2021. URL: https://www.paho.org/en/topics/chemical-safety#:~:text=The%202021%20data%20addendum%20estimates,exposure%20and%20resulting%20cardiovascular%20diseases.

[35] Agarwal P, Goyal A, Vaishnav RJ. Chemical hazards in pharmaceutical industry: an overview. Asian J Pharm Clin Res 2018;11:27-35.

[36] Bhusnure O, Dongare R, Gholve S, Giram PJ. Chemical hazards and safety management in pharmaceutical industry. J Pharm Res 2018;12(3):357-69.

[37] Hamsan H, Ho YB, Zaidon SZ, Hashim Z, Saari N, Karami A. Occurrence of commonly used pesticides in personal air samples and their associated health risk among paddy farmers. Sci Total Environ 2017;603:381-9.

[38] Meyer A, Sandler DP, Beane Freeman LE, Hofmann JN, Parks CG. Pesticide exposure and risk of rheumatoid arthritis among licensed male pesticide applicators in the agricultural health study. Environ Health Perspect 2017;125(7):077010.

[39] Gibb HJ, Lees PS, Pinsky PF, Rooney BC. Lung cancer among workers in chromium chemical production. Am J Industr Med 2000;38(2):115-26.

[40] Wong JY, Vermeulen R, Dai Y, Hu W, Martin WK, Warren SH, et al. Elevated urinary mutagenicity among those exposed to bituminous coal combustion emissions or diesel engine exhaust. Environ Molecul Mutagenesis 2021;62(8):458-70.

[41] Havet N, Penot A, Morelle M, Perrier L, Charbotel B, Fervers B. Varied exposure to carcinogenic, mutagenic, and reprotoxic (CMR) chemicals in occupational settings in France. Int Arch Occup Environ Health 2017;90(2):227-41.

[42] van Rooy FG, Rooyackers JM, Prokop M, Houba R, Smit LA, Heederik DJ. Bronchiolitis obliterans syndrome in chemical workers producing diacetyl for food flavorings. Am J Respir Crit Care Med 2007;176(5):498-504.

[43] Parks CG, Walitt BT, Pettinger M, Chen JC, de Roos AJ, Hunt J, et al. Insecticide use and risk of rheumatoid arthritis and systemic lupus erythematosus in the Women's Health Initiative Observational Study. Arthritis Care Res (Hoboken) 2011;63(2):184-94.

[44] Hu R, Huang X, Huang J, Li Y, Zhang C, Yin Y, et al. Long- and short-term health effects of pesticide exposure: a cohort study from China. PLoS One 2015;10(6):e0128766.
[45] Jindal BB, Sharma RJC, Materials B. The effect of nanomaterials on properties of geopolymers derived from industrial by-products: A state-of-the-art review. Constr Build Materials 2020;252:119028.
[46] Gajanan K, Tijare SN. Applications of nanomaterials. Materials Today Proceed 2018;5(1):1093-6.
[47] Gaines LGT. Historical and current usage of per- and polyfluoroalkyl substances (PFAS): A literature review. Am J Ind Med 2023;66(5):353-78.
[48] Glüge J, Scheringer M, Cousins IT, DeWitt JC, Goldenman G, Herzke D, et al. An overview of the uses of per-and polyfluoroalkyl substances (PFAS). Environ Sci Processes Impacts 2020;22(12):2345-73.
[49] Pettinari C, Marchetti F, Mosca N, Tosi G, Drozdov AJPI. Application of metal–organic frameworks. Polymer Int 2017;66(6):731-44.
[50] Czaja AU, Trukhan N, Müller UJCSR. Industrial applications of metal–organic frameworks. Chem Soc Rev 2009;38(5):1284-93.
[51] Yang H, Hitchcock E, Haldeman S, Swanson N, Lu ML, Choi B, et al. Workplace psychosocial and organizational factors for neck pain in workers in the United States. Am J Ind Med 2016;59(7):549-60.
[52] Battams S, Roche AM, Fischer JA, Lee NK, Cameron J, Kostadinov V. Workplace risk factors for anxiety and depression in male-dominated industries: a systematic review. Health Psychol Behav Med 2014;2(1):983-1008.
[53] Bonde JPE. Psychosocial factors at work and risk of depression: a systematic review of the epidemiological evidence. Occupat Environ Med 2008;65(7):438-45.
[54] Wilkinson RG, Marmot M. Social determinants of health: The solid facts. Geneva: World Health Organization, 2003.
[55] Wetterholm M, Turkiewicz A, Stigmar K, Hubertsson J, Englund MJAo. The rate of joint replacement in osteoarthritis depends on the patient's socioeconomic status: A cohort study of 71,380 patients. Acta Orthopaedica 2016;87(3):245-51.
[56] Peckham TK, Baker MG, Camp JE, Kaufman JD, Seixas NS. Creating a future for occupational health. Ann Work Expo Health 2017;61(1):3-15.
[57] Quick JC, Henderson DF. Occupational stress: Preventing suffering, enhancing wellbeing. Int J Environ Res Public Health 2016;13(5):459.

Chapter 4

How combined PFAS (per- and polyfluoroalkyl substances) and metals may contribute to chronic obstructive pulmonary disease

Aderonke Ayodele, MS
and Emmanuel Obeng-Gyasi*, PhD, MPH
Department of Built Environment and Environmental Health and Disease Laboratory, North Carolina A&T State University, Greensboro, North Carolina, United States of America

Abstract

This chapter explores the combined impact of PFAS (per- and polyfluoroalkyl substances) and heavy metals on respiratory health, focusing on their potential synergistic or additive effects. Evidence suggests that co-exposure to these contaminants may exacerbate pulmonary inflammation, oxidative stress, and lung injury. Studies indicate that PFAS and heavy metals, both known for their persistence and bioaccumulation in the environment, can disrupt immune responses, increase susceptibility to respiratory infections, and contribute to the development and exacerbation of COPD (chronic obstructive pulmonary disease). Given the limited research on the joint effects of PFAS and metals, this paper aims to fill the knowledge gap by providing insights into their interactive effects on respiratory health. It underscores the importance of regulatory measures to limit emissions of these contaminants and public health initiatives to reduce exposure.

---

* *Correspondence:* Emmanuel Obeng-Gyasi, PhD, MPH, Department of Built Environment and Environmental Health and Disease Laboratory, North Carolina A&T State University, Greensboro, NC 27411, United States of America. Email: eobenggyasi@ncat.edu

In: Public Health: Understanding the Impact of Environmental Pollutants
Editors: Emmanuel Obeng-Gyasi and Joav Merrick
ISBN: 979-8-89530-579-9
© 2025 Nova Science Publishers, Inc.

By addressing the combined impact of PFAS and metals, effective strategies can be developed to protect respiratory health and mitigate the risks associated with environmental pollutants.

Introduction

Environmental factors play a significant role in respiratory health, influencing both the onset and exacerbation of respiratory conditions. Several key environmental factors have been implicated in respiratory health issues such as climate change (1,2), air pollution (3, 4), occupational exposures (5, 6), indoor air quality (7, 8), and in some cases allergens (9), and respiratory infections (10, 11). According to Nishida and Yatera (12), ambient and occupational pollutants are implicated in various lung and respiratory diseases. Eguiluz-Gracia et al. (13) further emphasized that air pollution and climate change significantly impact respiratory health, with allergic rhinitis and asthma being common issues in Western countries. Researchers have also observed that the intersection of environmental, socioeconomic, and genetic factors can influence respiratory health outcomes (14, 15).

Per- and polyfluoroalkyl substances (PFAS) as air pollutants

Traditional air pollutants such as particulate matter ($PM_{2.5}$ and PM_{10}), carbon monoxide, volatile organic compounds (VOCs), and polycyclic aromatic hydrocarbons have established associations with respiratory discomfort and diseases (12, 16-18). PFAS are classified as emerging air pollutants because of their widespread industrial use and persistence in the environment (19,20). PFAS are known to be associated with a wide variety of health issues/dysfunctions ranging from elevated cholesterol and liver enzyme levels (21) to cancers (e.g., endometrial, thyroid, and testicular cancers) (22). However, their effect on respiratory health is currently being studied (23, 24). Burbank and colleagues found an association between serum PFAS concentration and asthma exacerbations, and the correlation between perfluorooctanoic acid (PFOA) and asthma attacks was substantial in the adolescent age group (12 – 18 year olds) (25). In another study, exposure of human bronchial epithelial cells to varied concentrations of PFAS such as short-chain (perfluorobutanoic acid, perflurobutane sulfonic acid and GenX) or long-chain (PFOA and perfluorooctane sulfonic acid (PFOS) revealed that PFOA and PFOS either as standalone or in a mixture had a priming and activating effect on NLRP3 inflammasome which could potentially contribute to asthma/airway hyper-responsiveness (26).

Metals as air pollutants

On the other hand, heavy metals like lead, mercury, and cadmium, are also found in the environment and can harm respiratory health. Occupational exposure to metals is the most common source of metal (including heavy metals) toxicity. It increases the risk of respiratory clinical outcomes such as lung cancers, bronchial asthma, pneumoconiosis, and chronic obstructive pulmonary disease (COPD) (27,28). Lung cancer risk has also been associated with occupational exposure to nickel dust and hexavalent chromium according to a recent study by Behrens et al. (29).

Objectives of this review

COPD is a progressive lung disease characterized by airflow limitation, significantly impacting breathing and overall quality of life. Understanding the joint effects of PFAS and metals on respiratory health, including conditions like COPD, is crucial. Current research on the combined impact of these environmental contaminants on COPD is limited, with few epidemiological and mechanistic studies available. This review will explore how PFAS and metals interact to affect respiratory health, providing insights into their combined effects and implications for diseases like COPD.

PFAS: Ubiquitous environmental contaminants

PFAS (per- and polyfluoroalkyl substances) are pervasive environmental contaminants known for their widespread presence due to various industrial and consumer applications (30). These synthetic chemicals have been used in a variety of products, including firefighting foams, non-stick cookware, water-repellent fabrics, and food packaging, because of their resistance to heat, water, and oil. The unique chemical properties of PFAS, particularly their strong carbon-fluorine bonds, make them exceptionally durable and resistant to degradation. As a result, they are often referred to as "forever chemicals."

Despite their utility, the persistence of PFAS in the environment and their potential adverse health effects have raised significant concerns (31). These substances can accumulate in the human body and the environment over time, leading to bioaccumulation and biomagnification. PFAS have been detected in water, soil, and air around the world, including remote areas far from any direct sources of contamination. Their widespread presence is attributed to both direct emissions from manufacturing and the degradation of consumer products containing PFAS (32).

Exposure to PFAS has been linked to various health issues, including cancer, liver damage, immune system suppression, and developmental effects in children (33, 34). The potential for long-term health impacts has prompted increased scrutiny and regulatory efforts to manage and mitigate their impact. Governments and environmental agencies are working to establish limits for PFAS in drinking water and to phase out the use of certain PFAS in consumer products.

As scientific understanding of PFAS continues to evolve, efforts to address their environmental and health impacts are becoming more urgent. Research is ongoing to develop effective methods for detecting, removing, and destroying PFAS in the environment. Additionally, public awareness and advocacy are playing crucial roles in driving policy changes and promoting safer alternatives to PFAS in industrial and consumer applications (35).

Metals: Environmental presence and respiratory health impacts

Metals, including heavy metals like lead, mercury, and cadmium, are prevalent environmental contaminants that can have detrimental effects on respiratory health (36). These metals are introduced into the environment through various sources, including industrial processes, mining, smelting, fossil fuel combustion, and the improper disposal of metal-containing products. Their persistence in the environment and potential for bioaccumulation make them significant public health concerns.

Heavy metals are known for their toxicity even at low concentrations (37). Once released into the environment, they can contaminate air, water, and soil, leading to widespread exposure. Inhalation of metal particles or fumes is a primary route of exposure that directly impacts respiratory health

(38). For example, inhaling lead particles can cause respiratory issues, as well as systemic effects such as neurotoxicity and developmental problems in children. Mercury vapor inhalation can lead to respiratory irritation, lung damage, and long-term neurological effects (39). Cadmium, often released from industrial processes and cigarette smoke, is particularly harmful to the lungs and has been associated with COPD, lung cancer, and other respiratory illnesses (40).

The mechanisms by which heavy metals impact respiratory health are varied. They can induce oxidative stress, inflammation, and damage to lung tissues (41, 42). These processes can exacerbate existing respiratory conditions such as asthma and bronchitis and increase the risk of developing new respiratory illnesses. Children, the elderly, and individuals with preexisting respiratory conditions are particularly vulnerable to the harmful effects of metal exposure.

Efforts to mitigate the impact of heavy metals on respiratory health include regulatory measures to limit emissions, the promotion of cleaner industrial practices, and the proper disposal and recycling of metal-containing products. Public health initiatives focus on monitoring air quality, educating communities about the risks of metal exposure, and providing resources for reducing exposure in high-risk areas (43).

Ongoing research aims to better understand the health effects of heavy metals and develop strategies for reducing their presence in the environment. Advances in air filtration technologies, soil remediation techniques, and alternative materials that reduce the need for toxic metals are critical components of these efforts (44). By addressing the sources and impacts of metal contamination, society can work towards a healthier environment and reduce the burden of respiratory illnesses linked to heavy metal exposure.

Overview of chronic obstructive pulmonary disease (COPD)

COPD is a progressive lung disease characterized by airflow limitation, which significantly impacts breathing and overall quality of life. COPD encompasses two main conditions: chronic bronchitis and emphysema, both of which contribute to the obstruction of airflow and difficulties in breathing (45). Chronic bronchitis involves inflammation and narrowing of the bronchial tubes, leading to increased mucus production and persistent coughing. Emphysema, on the other hand, is characterized by damage to the alveoli (air sacs) in the lungs, which impairs the lungs' ability to exchange oxygen and carbon dioxide efficiently. The combination of these conditions results in the hallmark symptoms of COPD: shortness of breath, chronic cough, wheezing, and frequent respiratory infections (46).

The primary cause of COPD is long-term exposure to irritants that damage the lungs and airways. The most significant risk factor is cigarette smoking, accounting for the majority of COPD cases. However, non-smokers can also develop COPD due to exposure to secondhand smoke, air pollution, occupational dust and chemicals, and genetic factors such as alpha-1 antitrypsin deficiency (47).

The progression of COPD varies among individuals but generally worsens over time. As the disease advances, everyday activities such as walking, climbing stairs, and even dressing can become challenging. The impact on quality of life is substantial, often leading to physical limitations, social isolation, and emotional distress (48).

Diagnosis of COPD typically involves spirometry, a test that measures lung function by assessing the volume and speed of air a person can exhale. Additional tests, such as chest X-rays and CT scans, may be used to assess lung damage and rule out other conditions. Early detection and management are crucial to slowing the progression of COPD and improving the quality of life for those affected (49).

Management of COPD includes a combination of lifestyle changes, medications, and pulmonary rehabilitation (50). Smoking cessation is the most effective intervention to prevent the progression of COPD. Medications, such as bronchodilators and corticosteroids, help to relieve symptoms and reduce inflammation. Pulmonary rehabilitation programs provide exercise training, nutritional advice, and education to help patients manage their condition and maintain their independence (51).

Despite the chronic nature of COPD, advancements in treatment and increased awareness of the disease offer hope for better outcomes. Ongoing research aims to develop new therapies and improve existing ones, with a focus on reducing symptoms, preventing exacerbations, and ultimately enhancing the quality of life for individuals living with COPD.

Interaction of PFAS and metals in promoting chronic obstructive pulmonary disease

The interaction of PFAS (per- and polyfluoroalkyl substances) and metals in the environment may significantly promote COPD. Both PFAS and metals are persistent environmental contaminants known to have adverse health effects, particularly on the respiratory system. When these substances coexist in the environment, their combined impact can exacerbate health conditions and contribute to the development and progression of COPD (52-54).

PFAS are synthetic chemicals widely used in various industrial and consumer products due to their heat, water, and oil resistance. They are known for their persistence in the environment and potential to bioaccumulate in living organisms. PFAS exposure has been linked to several health issues, including respiratory problems. These chemicals can induce inflammation, oxidative stress, and immune system dysfunction, all of which are contributing factors to respiratory diseases such as COPD (26, 55).

Metals, particularly heavy metals like lead, mercury, and cadmium, are also prevalent environmental contaminants with known toxicity. Exposure to heavy metals can occur through various routes, including inhalation of contaminated air. Heavy metals can damage lung tissues, induce oxidative stress, and cause chronic inflammation (56). These effects are directly associated with the development and exacerbation of COPD.

When PFAS and heavy metals coexist in the environment, their combined effects on respiratory health can be synergistic. For instance, both PFAS and metals can induce oxidative stress, leading to an overproduction of reactive oxygen species (ROS) and subsequent damage to lung cells. This oxidative damage can impair lung function and contribute to the chronic inflammation characteristic of COPD. Additionally, both contaminants can disrupt immune responses, making the lungs more susceptible to infections and exacerbations of COPD (57, 58).

Furthermore, the co-exposure to PFAS and heavy metals may enhance the bioavailability and toxicity of each other. For example, PFAS can alter the absorption and distribution of metals in the body, potentially increasing their toxic effects on the lungs. Similarly, metals can affect the metabolism and elimination of PFAS, leading to prolonged exposure and greater cumulative damage to the respiratory system (59).

The interaction of PFAS and heavy metals in the environment can have significant and synergistic effects on respiratory health, particularly in the development and progression of COPD. Both PFAS and heavy metals independently trigger inflammatory pathways, but their combined presence can lead to a heightened activation of pro-inflammatory cytokines and chemokines, exacerbating chronic inflammation in the lungs and accelerating COPD progression (60, 61). This inflammation is further compounded by their interference with normal lung repair mechanisms (62,63). Both contaminants can impair the regeneration of damaged epithelial cells and extracellular matrix components, leading to structural changes in the airways and alveoli that are characteristic of COPD.

Additionally, PFAS and metals may disrupt mucociliary clearance, affecting the function of cilia and mucus production in the respiratory tract. This disruption can result in the accumulation of pollutants and pathogens in the lungs, increasing the risk of respiratory infections and exacerbations of COPD. Exposure to these contaminants can also lead to epigenetic modifications, such as DNA methylation and histone acetylation, which alter the expression of genes involved in lung function and immune responses, thereby contributing to the development and progression of COPD (64-66).

The oxidative stress generated by PFAS and metals is another critical factor. While both independently produce reactive oxygen species (ROS), their combined exposure can create a more significant oxidative burden, overwhelming antioxidant defenses and resulting in extensive lung tissue damage and inflammation. Moreover, PFAS, known as endocrine disruptors, and heavy metals, which can interfere with hormonal balance, can together affect the regulation of hormones crucial for lung health, such as glucocorticoids, potentially worsening COPD symptoms (67, 68).

Finally, both PFAS and heavy metals can hinder the body's natural detoxification processes (69, 70). This impairment leads to the accumulation of toxic substances in lung tissues, further contributing to respiratory damage and the progression of COPD. The combined effects of these contaminants create a complex and multifaceted challenge for respiratory health, emphasizing the need for comprehensive strategies to mitigate their impact.

Conclusion

Research on the combined impact of PFAS and metals on respiratory health is still emerging, but the existing evidence highlights the need for a comprehensive approach to address environmental contaminants. Regulatory measures to limit emissions of both PFAS and heavy metals and public health initiatives to reduce exposure are critical steps in mitigating their impact on respiratory health and preventing COPD.

Understanding the interaction between PFAS and metals is essential for developing effective strategies to protect public health. Ongoing research aims to elucidate the mechanisms of their combined toxicity and identify interventions to reduce the risk of COPD and other respiratory diseases associated with environmental contaminants. By addressing these interactions, we can work towards a healthier environment and improve respiratory health outcomes for affected populations.

Acknowledgments

Conceptualization, E.O.-G.; methodology, E.O.-G; formal analysis, A.A., E.O.-G..; investigation, A.A., E.O.-G.; resources, E.O.-G.; data curation, E.O.-G.; writing—original draft preparation, A.A., and E.O.-G.; writing—review and editing, A.A., E.O.-G; supervision, E.O.-G.; project administration, E.O.-G.; funding acquisition, E.O.-G. All authors have read and agreed to the published version of the manuscript. Funding: Research reported in this publication was supported by the National Institute of General Medical Sciences of the National Institutes of Health under Award Number R16GM149473. The content is solely the responsibility of the authors and does not necessarily represent the official views of the National Institutes of Health.

References

[1] D'Amato G, Chong-Neto HJ, Monge Ortega OP, Vitale C, Ansotegui I, Rosario N, et al. The effects of climate change on respiratory allergy and asthma induced by pollen and mold allergens. Allergy 2020;75(9):2219-28.

[2] Aguilera R, Corringham T, Gershunov A, Benmarhnia T. Wildfire smoke impacts respiratory health more than fine particles from other sources: observational evidence from Southern California. Nat Commun 2021;12(1):1493.

[3] Chatkin J, Correa L, Santos U. External environmental pollution as a risk factor for asthma. Clin Rev Allergy Immunol 2022;62(1):72-89.

[4] Jainonthee C, Wang YL, Chen CWK, Jainontee K. Air pollution-related respiratory diseases and associated environmental factors in Chiang Mai, Thailand, in 2011-2020. Trop Med Infect Dis 2022;7(11):341.

[5] Archangelidi O, Sathiyajit S, Consonni D, Jarvis D, Matteis SD. Cleaning products and respiratory health outcomes in occupational cleaners: A systematic review and meta-analysis. O Occup Environ Med 2020:oemed-2020-106776.

[6] Amoabeng Nti AA, Arko-Mensah J, Botwe PK, Dwomoh D, Kwarteng L, Takyi SA, et al. Effect of particulate matter exposure on respiratory health of e-waste

workers at Agbogbloshie, Accra, Ghana. Int J Environ Res Public Health 2020;17(9):3042.

[7] Wolkoff P, Azuma K, Carrer P. Health, work performance, and risk of infection in office-like environments: The role of indoor temperature, air humidity, and ventilation. Int J Hyg Environ Health 2021;233:113709.

[8] Rosário Filho NA, Urrutia-Pereira M, D'Amato G, Cecchi L, Ansotegui IJ, Galán C, et al. Air pollution and indoor settings. World Allergy Organ J 2021;14(1):100499.

[9] Lam HCY, Jarvis D, Fuertes E. Interactive effects of allergens and air pollution on respiratory health: A systematic review. Sci Total Environ 2021;757:143924.

[10] Qu G, Li X, Hu L, Jiang G. An imperative need for research on the role of environmental factors in transmission of novel coronavirus (COVID-19). Environ Sci Technol 2020;54(7):3730-2.

[11] Chen W, Zhang N, Wei J, Yen H-L, Li Y. Short-range airborne route dominates exposure of respiratory infection during close contact. Build Environment 2020;176:106859.

[12] Nishida C, Yatera K. The impact of ambient environmental and occupational pollution on respiratory diseases. Int J Environ Res Public Health 2022;19(5):2788.

[13] Eguiluz-Gracia I, Mathioudakis AG, Bartel S, Vijverberg SJH, Fuertes E, Comberiati P, et al. The need for clean air: The way air pollution and climate change affect allergic rhinitis and asthma. Allergy 2020;75(9):2170-84.

[14] Kunachowicz D, Ściskalska M, Kepinska M. Modulatory effect of lifestyle-related, environmental and genetic factors on paraoxonase-1 activity: A review. Int J Environ Res Public Health 2023;20(4):2813.

[15] Liang H, Zhou X, Zhu Y, Li D, Jing D, Su X, et al. Association of outdoor air pollution, lifestyle, genetic factors with the risk of lung cancer: A prospective cohort study. Environ Res 2023;218:114996.

[16] Domingo JL, Rovira J. Effects of air pollutants on the transmission and severity of respiratory viral infections. Environ Res 2020;187:109650.

[17] Obeng GM, Aram SA, Agyei D, Saalidong BM. Exposure to particulate matter (PM2.5) and volatile organic compounds (VOCs), and self-reported health symptoms among fish smokers: A case study in the Western Region of Ghana. PLoS One 2023;18(3):e0283438.

[18] Alves C, Evtyugina M, Vicente E, Vicente A, Rienda IC, de la Campa AS, et al. PM2.5 chemical composition and health risks by inhalation near a chemical complex. J Environ Sci 2023;124:860-74.

[19] Al Amin M, Sobhani Z, Liu Y, Dharmaraja R, Chadalavada S, Naidu R, et al. Recent advances in the analysis of per- and polyfluoroalkyl substances (PFAS): A review. Environ Technol Innovat 2020;19:100879.

[20] Abunada Z, Alazaiza MYD, Bashir MJK. An overview of per- and polyfluoroalkyl substances (PFAS) in the environment: Source, fate, risk and regulations. Water 2020;12(12):3590.

[21] Boyd RI, Ahmad S, Singh R, Fazal Z, Prins GS, Madak Erdogan Z, et al. Toward a mechanistic understanding of poly- and perfluoroalkylated substances and cancer. Cancers 2022;14(12):2919.
[22] Seyyedsalehi MS, Boffetta P. Per- and poly-fluoroalkyl substances (PFAS) exposure and risk of kidney, liver, and testicular cancers: A systematic review and meta-analysis. Med Lav 2023;114(5):e2023040.
[23] Kvalem HE, Nygaard UC, Lødrup Carlsen KC, Carlsen KH, Haug LS, Granum B. Perfluoroalkyl substances, airways infections, allergy and asthma related health outcomes – implications of gender, exposure period and study design. Environ Int 2020;134:105259.
[24] Shi S, Ding Y, Wu B, Hu P, Chen M, Dong N, et al. Association of perfluoroalkyl substances with pulmonary function in adolescents (NHANES 2007–2012). Environ Sci Pollut Res Int 2023;30(18):53948-61.
[25] Burbank AJ, Fry RC, Keet CA. Associations between serum per- and polyfluoroalkyl substances and asthma morbidity in the National Health and Nutrition Examination Survey (2003-18). J Allergy Clin Immunol Glob 2023;2(2):100078.
[26] Dragon J, Hoaglund M, Badireddy AR, Nielsen G, Schlezinger J, Shukla A. Perfluoroalkyl substances (PFAS) affect inflammation in lung cells and tissues. Int J Mol Sci 2023;24(10):8539.
[27] Vanka KS, Shukla S, Gomez HM, James C, Palanisami T, Williams K, et al. Understanding the pathogenesis of occupational coal and silica dust-associated lung disease. Eur Respir Rev 2022;31(165).
[28] Mozaffari S, Heibati B, Jaakkola MS, Lajunen TK, Kalteh S, Alimoradi H, et al. Effects of occupational exposures on respiratory health in steel factory workers. Front Public Health 2023;11:1082874.
[29] Behrens T, Ge C, Vermeulen R, Kendzia B, Olsson A, Schüz J, et al. Occupational exposure to nickel and hexavalent chromium and the risk of lung cancer in a pooled analysis of case-control studies (SYNERGY). Int J Cancer 2023;152(4):645-60.
[30] Garg S, Kumar P, Mishra V, Guijt R, Singh P, Dumée LF, et al. A review on the sources, occurrence and health risks of per-/poly-fluoroalkyl substances (PFAS) arising from the manufacture and disposal of electric and electronic products. J Water Process Eng 2020;38:101683.
[31] Cousins IT, DeWitt JC, Glüge J, Goldenman G, Herzke D, Lohmann R, et al. The high persistence of PFAS is sufficient for their management as a chemical class. Environ Sci Process Impacts 2020;22(12):2307-12.
[32] Liddie JM, Schaider LA, Sunderland EM. Sociodemographic factors are associated with the abundance of PFAS sources and detection in US community water systems. Environ Sci Technol 2023;57(21):7902-12.
[33] Ehrlich V, Bil W, Vandebriel R, Granum B, Luijten M, Lindeman B, et al. Consideration of pathways for immunotoxicity of per-and polyfluoroalkyl substances (PFAS). Environ Health 2023;22(1):19.
[34] Agency for Toxic Substances and Disease Registry (ATSDR). Per-and polyfluoroalkyl substances (PFAS) and your health. Atlanta, GA: ATSDR, 2020.

[35] Glenn G, Shogren R, Jin X, Orts W, Hart-Cooper W, Olson L. Per-and polyfluoroalkyl substances and their alternatives in paper food packaging. Compr Rev Food Sci Food Saf 2021;20(3):2596-625.
[36] Obeng-Gyasi E. Sources of lead exposure in West Africa. Sci 2022;4(3):33.
[37] Lanphear BP, Rauch S, Auinger P, Allen RW, Hornung RW. Low-level lead exposure and mortality in US adults: A population-based cohort study. Lancet Public Health 2018;3(4):e177-84.
[38] Blanuša M, Telišman S, Hršak J, Fugaš M, Prpić-Majić D, Šarić M. Assessment of exposure to lead and cadmium through air and food in inhabitants of Zagreb. Arh Hig Rada Toksikol 1991;42(3):257-66.
[39] Kim K, Park H. Association of mercury exposure with the serum high-sensitivity C-reactive protein level in Korean adults. Front Public Health 2023;11:1062741.
[40] Ganguly K, Levänen B, Palmberg L, Åkesson A, Lindén A. Cadmium in tobacco smokers: A neglected link to lung disease? Eur Respir Rev 2018;27(147):170122.
[41] Obeng-Gyasi E. Lead exposure and oxidative stress—A life course approach in US adults. Toxics 2018;6(3):42.
[42] Valko M, Morris H, Cronin M. Metals, toxicity and oxidative stress. Curr Med Chem 2005;12(10):1161-208.
[43] Geiger A, Cooper J. Overview of airborne metals regulations, exposure limits, health effects, and contemporary research. Portland, OR: Environmental Protection Agency, 2010:1-56.
[44] Gondal A. Nanotechnology advancement in the elimination of chemical toxins from air spectrums. Int J Environ Sci Technol (Tehran) 2023;20(11):12775-92.
[45] Rennard SI. COPD: overview of definitions, epidemiology, and factors influencing its development. Chest 1998;113(4):235S-41S.
[46] Agusti A, Soriano JB. COPD as a systemic disease. COPD 2008;5(2):133-8.
[47] Soriano JB, Rodríguez-Roisin R. Chronic obstructive pulmonary disease overview: Epidemiology, risk factors, and clinical presentation. Proc Am Thorac Soc 2011;8(4):363-7.
[48] Cruz J, Marques A, Figueiredo D. Impacts of COPD on family carers and supportive interventions: a narrative review. Health Soc Care Commun 2017;25(1):11-25.
[49] Csikesz NG, Gartman EJ. New developments in the assessment of COPD: early diagnosis is key. Int J Chron Obstruct Pulmon Dis 2014;9:277-86.
[50] Izquierdo JL, Morena D, González Y, Paredero JM, Pérez B, Graziani D, et al. Clinical management of COPD in a real-world setting. A big data analysis. Arch Bronconeumol (Engl Ed) 2021;57(2):94-100.
[51] Vogelmeier CF, Roman-Rodriguez M, Singh D, Han MK, Rodriguez-Roisin R, Ferguson GT. Goals of COPD treatment: focus on symptoms and exacerbations. Respir Med 2020;166:105938.
[52] Boafo YS, Mostafa S, Obeng-Gyasi E. Association of combined metals and PFAS with cardiovascular disease risk. Toxics 2023;11(12):979.
[53] Haruna I, Obeng-Gyasi E. Association of combined per-and polyfluoroalkyl substances and metals with chronic kidney disease. Int J Environ Res Public Health 2024;21(4):468.

[54] Bashir T, Obeng-Gyasi E. The association of combined per-and polyfluoroalkyl substances and metals with allostatic load using Bayesian Kernel Machine Regression. Diseases 2023;11(1):52.
[55] Wielsøe M, Long M, Ghisari M, Bonefeld-Jørgensen EC. Perfluoroalkylated substances (PFAS) affect oxidative stress biomarkers in vitro. Chemosphere 2015;129:239-45.
[56] Anka AU, Usman AB, Kaoje AN, Kabir RM, Bala A, Kazem Arki M, et al. Potential mechanisms of some selected heavy metals in the induction of inflammation and autoimmunity. Eur J Inflam 2022;20:1721727X221122719.
[57] Lopez-Espinosa M-J, Carrizosa C, Luster MI, Margolick JB, Costa O, Leonardi GS, et al. Perfluoroalkyl substances and immune cell counts in adults from the Mid-Ohio Valley (USA). Environ Int 2021;156:106599.
[58] Wang M, Xia W, Zeng Q, Zhang W, Qian X, Bao S, et al. Associations between prenatal and postnatal lead exposure and preschool children humoral and cellular immune responses. Ecotoxicol Environ Saf 2021;207:111536.
[59] Tsaioun K, Blaauboer BJ, Hartung T. Evidence-based absorption, distribution, metabolism, excretion (ADME) and its interplay with alternative toxicity methods. ALTEX 2016;33(4):343-58.
[60] Zhang L, Louie A, Rigutto G, Guo H, Zhao Y, Ahn S, et al. A systematic evidence map of chronic inflammation and immunosuppression related to per-and polyfluoroalkyl substance (PFAS) exposure. Environ Res 2023;220:115188.
[61] Dobrakowski M, Kasperczyk A, Pawlas N, Birkner E, Hudziec E, Chwalińska E, et al. Association between subchronic and chronic lead exposure and levels of antioxidants and chemokines. Int Arch Occup Environ Health 2016;89:1077-85.
[62] Wei W, Wu X, Bai Y, Li G, Feng Y, Meng H, et al. Lead exposure and its interactions with oxidative stress polymorphisms on lung function impairment: Results from a longitudinal population-based study. Environ Res 2020;187:109645.
[63] Sørli JB, Låg M, Ekeren L, Perez-Gil J, Haug LS, Da Silva E, et al. Per-and polyfluoroalkyl substances (PFASs) modify lung surfactant function and pro-inflammatory responses in human bronchial epithelial cells. Toxicol In Vitro 2020;62:104656.
[64] Khalid M, Abdollahi M. Epigenetic modifications associated with pathophysiological effects of lead exposure. J Environ Sci Health C Environ Carcinog Ecotoxicol Rev 2019;37(4):235-87.
[65] Cuomo D, Foster MJ, Threadgill D. Systemic review of genetic and epigenetic factors underlying differential toxicity to environmental lead (Pb) exposure. Environ Sci Pollut Res Int 2022;29(24):35583-98.
[66] Kim S, Thapar I, Brooks BW. Epigenetic changes by per-and polyfluoroalkyl substances (PFAS). Environ Pollut 2021;279:116929.
[67] Rickard BP, Rizvi I, Fenton SE. Per-and poly-fluoroalkyl substances (PFAS) and female reproductive outcomes: PFAS elimination, endocrine-mediated effects, and disease. Toxicology 2022;465:153031.

[68] Javorac D, Baralić K, Marić Đ, Mandić-Rajčević S, Đukić-Ćosić D, Bulat Z, et al. Exploring the endocrine disrupting potential of lead through benchmark modelling–study in humans. Environ Pollut 2023;316:120428.
[69] Genuis S, Birkholz D, Ralitsch M, Thibault N. Human detoxification of perfluorinated compounds. Public Health 2010;124(7):367-75.
[70] Carocci A, Catalano A, Lauria G, Sinicropi MS, Genchi G. Lead toxicity, antioxidant defense and environment. Rev Environ Contam Toxicol 2016;238:45-67.

Chapter 5

A review on the potential lead pollution in domestic water use in the State of Mississippi

William Dodoo Sackey[1], MPH
and Emmanuel Obeng-Gyasi[2,3,*], MPH, PhD

[1]Jackson State University, Department of Public Health, Jackson Medical Mall, Jackson, Mississippi, United States of America
[2]Department of Built Environment, North Carolina A&T State University, Greensboro, North Carolina, United States of America
[3]Environmental Health and Disease Laboratory, North Carolina A&T State University, Greensboro, North Carolina, United States of America

Abstract

Not so long ago, the city of Jackson, Mississippi, was overwhelmed by severe water challenges following the failure of the city's largest water treatment plant. This led to acute water shortage, with most residents being unable to access clean tap water. Several communities with running tap water had to subject such water to boiling to perform domestic tasks such as bathing or cleaning, as such water was generally unsafe and consisted of dirt and soil sediments. The breakdown in the water treatment plant is largely attributed to severe storms, which led to the flooding of the Pearl River, which serves as the source of the Jackson water system. Although the storms and floods were a significant factor, the Jackson water system has long been subjected to a culture of neglect and poor maintenance. The poor maintenance culture poses a significant public health threat and causes the old, rusty water

---

* *Correspondence:* Emmanuel Obeng-Gyasi, MPH, PhD, Department of Built Environment and Environmental Health and Disease Laboratory, North Carolina A&T State University, Greensboro, NC 27411, United States of America. Email: eobengyasi@ncat.edu

In: Public Health: Understanding the Impact of Environmental Pollutants
Editors: Emmanuel Obeng-Gyasi and Joav Merrick
ISBN: 979-8-89530-579-9
© 2025 Nova Science Publishers, Inc.

pipelines to leach lead over time, and this has severe health implications. This paper presents a literature review on the potential for lead pollution in domestic water use within the southern state of Mississippi and highlights existing legislation from agencies such as the United States Environmental Protection Agency (EPA), which exist to address the problem. This chapter further discusses some potential health implications of lead toxicity, such as elevated blood pressure, renal impairments, and even death in very severe cases.

Introduction

The largest water treatment plant in Jackson, Mississippi, broke down on 29th August 2022, affecting 160,000 persons, schools, hospitals as well as fire stations, leaving them with no safe drinking water, and in several situations, no water services in any of these communities (1). The urban water challenges in Jackson expose the fragility and vulnerability of the water system to flooding resulting from climate change (2). The crises occurred primarily because continuous rainfall resulted in the flooding of the Pearl River watershed where the OB Curtis water treatment plant is situated, placing the pump out of order (2).

The fact remains that globally, water systems are under constraints due to economic advancements, population increments, urbanization, and, in recent times, changes in climate variability (3). Even though concerns about the source, pureness, and safety of water are often considered a problem associated with low-income countries, events that ultimately led to a state of emergency in Jackson, Mississippi, in 2022 bring to bear the problems that result from poor water infrastructure (4). In situations where water infrastructure fails because of deterioration or other reasons, the physical stability of the system is broken down and compromises barriers to potential contamination (5).

This review aims to identify the potential for lead (Pb) contamination in domestic water usage in the state of Mississippi from a public health perspective, highlight regulatory measures that exist to remedy the situation, and identify some health challenges that may result from Pb intake. The review concludes by providing alternative solutions to Pb water pipes and provides recommendations and future perspectives.

Literature review

The Bureau of Public Water Supply, under the Mississippi State Department of Health, indicates that it supplies safe drinking water to citizens of Mississippi by strictly enacting the provisions of the Federal and State Safe Drinking Water Act (6). The Safe Drinking Water Act is a law put in place to safeguard the quality of drinking water in the United States (7). Through this law, the EPA indicates that it has the authority to provide basic standards for tap water protection and ensure that public water system operators conform to these standards.

Groundwater in Jackson, Mississippi

Jackson is a city central to the Jackson Metropolitan Statistical Area. It comprises counties such as Hinds, Madison, Copiah, Simpson, and Rankin (8). The Ross Barnett Reservoir, which covers an area of 52 square miles, is the primary water source for the Jackson Water System and is managed by the Pearl River Valley Water Supply District (8).

The water situation in Jackson has recently made news headlines as a significant potential environmental challenge affecting the inhabitants' public health and welfare (9). However, this issue is not new, as similar consciousness around Pb contamination occurred during the Flint, Michigan Pb crisis of 2014-2019. Indeed, during these developments in Flint, Michigan, the inhabitants of Jackson discovered that the Mississippi State Department of Health analyzed water samples from a section of Jackson homes and found that many samples had Pb levels above guidelines established by the EPA (10). The Mississippi State Department of Health (MSDH), in January 2016, indicated that 22% of water samples evaluated in June 2015 contained Pb levels beyond the federal action level of 15 ppb (11). Indeed, the MSDH between 2009 and 2015 documented 3083 children with elevated levels of Pb in their blood (11).

Lead pollution

Pb is a heavy metal that occurs in abundance within the Earth's crust, with an average concentration of approximately 14 parts per million by weight, or about 1 part per million by moles (12). Pb is a bluish-grey metal with a low melting point that can be easily shaped and forms alloys with other metals (13). Pb uptake and exposure have been linked to factors such as pollution from industrialization, paint containing Pb traces, plumbing infrastructure in old buildings, soil with Pb residues, dietary factors, and social issues such as low-income levels, stress, and racial disparities (14).

Pb seeps into drinking water from corroded service pipes (15). Pb poisoning usually occurs through food or drinking Pb-contaminated water (16) and poses a considerable threat to human health due to the release of inflammatory mediators in tissues (17). The daily maximum intake of Pb is 1.0ug/g. However, the intake of Pb, even at such low levels, is considered hazardous to human health (16).

Health implications of lead poisoning

Toxicity from Pb is severe for human health (13). Pb induces oxidative stress due to the disruption in the regeneration of glutathione, a critical antioxidant (13). Pb may also result in hemolytic anemia because of cellular membrane disruption from lipid peroxidation (13). Increased levels of Pb in the blood affect behavior, cognitive ability, delays in puberty, postnatal growth retardation, and reduces hearing abilities in children and infants (18). Pb leads to central nervous system, kidney, cardiovascular as well as fertility problems in adults (18). Being exposed to Pb before and during pregnancy can have harmful effects (19) Pb, which accumulates in bones due to its 30-year half-life, can be released during pregnancy, particularly when blood calcium levels are low (19).

According to the United States Centers for Disease Control and Prevention (CDC), Mississippi accepted $300,000 from the CDC in fiscal year 2002 through a cooperative agreement to fund childhood Pb poisoning and surveillance programs (20). The CDC indicated that strategies adopted for the program include emphasizing blood testing and reporting, intensifying surveillance on blood Pb, and facilitating linkages to recommended services (20).

Regulations targeted at lead control

The United States Congress has enacted legislation explicitly addressing Pb contamination and exposure (21). The EPA regulates Pb contamination and manages hazardous events related to it by implementing and enforcing relevant environmental laws. These laws include the Toxic Substances Control Act, the Clean Air Act, and the Safe Drinking Water Act.

The Toxic Substances Control Act (1976) authorizes the EPA to demand reporting, testing, and record-keeping as well as place limitations on chemical substances, with the general exemption of food, pesticides, medications, and cosmetic products (22). The act focuses on manufacturing, importing, utilizing, and discarding chemicals such as Pb-based paint, asbestos, and polychlorinated biphenyls (22). The Clean Air Act refers to the federal legislation that controls air discharges emanating from mobile and stationary sources. It authorizes the EPA to implement National Ambient Air Quality Standards (NAAQS) to safeguard public health and control the release of hazardous pollutants from the air (23).

The Safe Drinking Water Act was originally established by Congress in 1974, to safeguard the public's healthy regulating the public drinking water supply of the nation and provides authorization to the United States EPA to establish national health-based benchmarks for drinking water (24). Pb in water is regulated jointly by the Clean Water Act as well as the Safe Water Act, and as indicated by the EPA, unless an entity is in procession of a National Pollution Discharge Elimination System Permit (NPDE), the Clean Water Act places restrictions on discharge of pollutants such as Pb into a United States Water body through a point source (21).

The Mississippi State Department of Health coordinates sampling of public water systems routinely per requirements of the Environmental Protection Agency and indicates that three (3) out of 160 water samples collected from January to June 2021 had Pb levels above the limits set by the EPA, which is 15 parts per billion (24).

The table below shows lead sample summary results from selected Public Water Systems (PWS) within the state of Mississippi.

Table 1. Lead summary results from sample public water systems in Mississippi from 2013-2019 (11)

County	Public Water System	Population Served	Sample Size	Beginning of Monitoring Period	End of Monitoring Period	90th Percentile
Bolivar	Boyle-Skene WA #3	1,373	10	1/1/13	12/31/15	4.6
Bolivar	Town of Merigold	552	10	1/1/15	12/31/17	5.2
Bolivar	Town of Benoit	500	10	1/1/15	12/31/17	8.1
Coahoma	Green Acres W/A South	260	5	1/1/15	12/31/17	3.1
Coahoma	Moore Bayou W/A #2	526	17	1/1/15	12/31/17	3.6
Coahoma	Coahoma Community College	2000	21	1/1/17	6/30/17	7
Humphreys	Town of Silver City	337	5	1/1/15	12/31/17	7.6
Leflore	City of Schlater	334	5	1/1/15	12/31/17	4.3
Panola	Plum Point Water System	126	5	1/1/17	12/31/17	5.5
Quitman County	Darling Water Association	300	5	1/1/17	12/31/17	4.5
Quitman County	Town of Crowder	700	10	1/1/17	12/31/19	29.2

Clinical manifestation of lead poisoning

Pb is an environmental pollutant, and regardless of the small amounts absorbed, increased exposure to Pb can result in accumulation in the human body and cause poisoning and toxicity (25). Pb accrues within the human body throughout life and damages cell parts such as lysosomes, mitochondria, and critical enzymes required for cell division and metabolism, leading to damage to DNA and morphological changes in the nucleus (26).

From a physiological perspective, Pb causes dysregulation of several organ systems, such as the renal, nervous, and hematologic systems (27). Anemia, which is one of the common outcomes from excessive Pb exposure, results from the inhibition of enzymes delta-Aminolaevulinic acid Dehydratase (ALAD), as well as ferro chelatase; these are critical enzymes that contribute to heme synthesis and leads to the formation of zinc protoporphyrin, a laboratory marker for Pb (28). Exposure to Pb can also damage the male reproductive system, and the damaging effects on the testes as well as the hypothalamic-pituitary-gonadal axis are believed to be the main pathway (26).

Pb poisoning in children is an important issue of public health significance in the United States and globally (29). There is an increasing rise in asymptomatic Pb poisoning among pediatric patients due to the universal presence of Pb in the environment as well as its sustained use for industrial purposes (27). Children who are less than six years of age are mostly at risk as it may result in impairments in their physical and mental growth (27).

The United States Centers for Disease Control and Prevention (CDC) indicates that conducting a blood test for Pb is the best means of determining Pb exposure in a child (21). The blood test is done by drawing a child's blood sample through a finger prick or venous blood draw (30) and provides an efficient means to monitor the Pb exposure risk. Table 2 indicates some clinical symptoms associated with Pb poisoning in various human organ systems.

Table 2. General clinical manifestations of Pb poisoning in human organs (18)

Human system/Organ	Clinical symptom
Eyes	Hallucinations Blindness Slurred Speech
Ears	Loss of hearing
Mouth	Blue line along the mouth
Liver	Jaundice Hemosiderosis Cholestasis Oxidative Stress (Lead induced)
Skin	Pallor
Reproductive Organs	Preterm birth Sperm dysfunctions Pregnancy complications
Abdomen	Pain Constipation Diarrhea Nausea
Central Nervous System	Headaches Memory Loss Coma

Methodology

The literature for our study was identified based on the PRISMA model, using keywords and searching relevant databases to select the most appropriate publications (see Figure 1). Google Scholar and PubMed databases were searched from 2014 to 2024. References of selected articles were also checked to find related articles. Selected articles were screened according to their suitability to meet set eligibility criteria which included search terms such as: ("lead (Pb) contamination" OR "lead (Pb) water contamination Mississippi", "heavy metal pollution" OR "heavy metal contamination Mississippi", "lead (Pb) water toxicity" OR "lead (Pb) water contamination Mississippi", lead (Pb) pollution OR lead (Pb) water pollution Jackson").

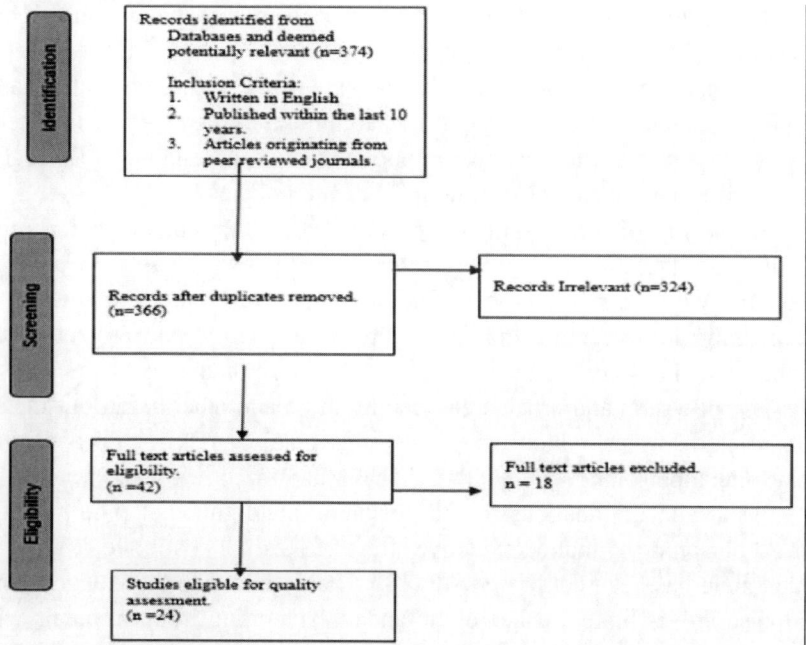

Figure 1. Prisma Flow diagram of the identification and selection of literature.

Discussion

Although the water management agencies in Mississippi have contributed to ensuring some degree of equity in the distribution of water, several challenges exist concerning Pb exposure risk. Results from the twenty-four assessed articles published in the last ten years were critically analyzed in this study and compared with previous literature. Similarities were evident regarding the dire environmental consequences of Pb and its potential to pollute domestic water sources. Previous literature (4, 5) has highlighted the impact of poor maintenance and infrastructural deficits in water systems, linking these factors to sources of Pb contamination in Mississippi. Additionally, previous incidents of Pb contamination, such as the crisis in Flint, Michigan, as explained by Rosner and colleagues (10), further justify the need for immediate action. The Flint, Michigan Pb contamination crisis underscored the severe risks associated with Pb exposure, particularly in vulnerable populations. This crisis not only exposed thousands of residents, including children, to toxic levels of Pb but also highlighted the broader social determinants of health. Factors such as socioeconomic status, racial disparities, and inadequate infrastructure played a significant role in exacerbating the situation. The crisis revealed how environmental hazards disproportionately affect marginalized communities, leading to long-term health consequences, loss of trust in public institutions, and a call for urgent reforms in water management and public health policies.

Our search of the literature also indicated that Pb contamination often results from the corrosion of service pipelines, which releases Pb particles into the water supply. These findings underscore the importance of maintaining infrastructure to prevent Pb contamination and protect public health (15). In addition, aged water distribution systems, as is the case in Mississippi's rural and urban areas, can leach Pb and other hazardous metals into drinking water, which may place households at risk for Pb and other heavy metal poisoning.

The health implications for Pb poisoning are significant. The potential for Pb poisoning to induce oxidative stress via disruptions in the renewal of glutathione has been confirmed (13, 18). The literature further suggests that Pb poisoning is linked to hemolytic anemia stemming from problems with the peroxidation of lipids (13). The effects of Pb poisoning are particularly dire in the case of pregnant women and young children, with Rees and colleagues (19) confirming that Pb accumulated in the bones of an expectant mother can be discharged during pregnancy, especially when there are low blood calcium levels.

In the case of young children, Boskabady and colleagues (18) confirmed that Pb poisoning can lead to cognitive deficits and behavioral problems in young children as it readily crosses the blood-brain barrier.

The available literature indicates that legislative provisions for regulating Pb exist in the United States, as established by the Environmental Protection Agency. Such legislative provisions include the Toxic Substances Control Act (1976), which authorizes the EPA to require reporting, testing, and record-keeping of potentially toxic substances and emphasizes the manufacturing, use, and disposal of chemicals such as Pb-based paint. Other existing legislation includes the Clean Air Act (1963), which focuses on controlling air discharges, and the Safe Drinking Water Act (1974), which primarily focuses on regulating public drinking water. Enforcement of these regulations is essential at all times, with a particular focus on areas inhabited by populations who have historically borne the brunt of environmental pollution. This targeted approach ensures that vulnerable communities are protected from the adverse health effects of Pb exposure.

The Mississippi State Department of Health is primarily responsible for local regulation of public drinking water and is involved in the coordination of sampling of public drinking water. Recently available literature suggested some level of Pb pollution, as water samples collected between January and June 2021 had Pb levels above acceptable limits set by the EPA (24). This contamination reflects the extent of the Pb pollution problem, which serves as a wake-up call for public health and environmental stakeholders to continuously monitor Pb levels in drinking water.

Conclusion and future perspectives

Heavy metal, and by extension Pb exposure, in principal cities such as Jackson, Mississippi, has made news headlines in recent years and is a wake-up call for immediate action. Recommendations for action include an overhaul of existing pipeline infrastructure and a replacement of Pb pipes with polyvinyl chloride pipes, which are generally considered safer and much more durable. State Agencies, such as the Mississippi State Department of Health, with support from the Environmental Protection Agency, should set guidelines within a workable time frame to replace Pb pipes and intensify surveillance on Pb levels through close collaboration.

Enforcement of federal and state policies banning the use of Pb pipes for domestic water distribution must be monitored. In addition, the use of alternative sustainable materials in the design of water pipelines must be explored.

Finally, public health efforts should be targeted at health education on the dangers of Pb exposure and pollution. The State Department of Health must intensify local collaborative efforts with primary care providers to integrate screening activities into routine health care activities for early detection and prevention of Pb poisoning. These recommendations may go a long way in addressing the challenge of Pb exposure within states such as Mississippi.

Acknowledgments

Conceptualization, W.D.S.; methodology, W.D.S., E.O.-G; formal analysis, W.D.S., investigation, W.D.S.; data curation, W.D.S.; writing—original draft preparation, W.D.S; writing—review and editing, W.D.S., E.O.-G. All authors have read and agreed to the published version of the manuscript. Funding: Obeng-Gyasi is funded by the National Institutes of Health under Award Number R16GM149473. He is also funded by the BCSP Foundation.

References

[1] Southern Poverty Law Center. History of Jackson, Mississippi, water crisis. Southern Poverty Law Center. URL: https://www.splcenter.org/news/2023/06/28/timeline-jackson-mississippi-water-problems.

[2] Meng Q. Urban water crisis causes significant public health diseases in Jackson, Mississippi USA: An initial study of geographic and racial health inequities. Sustainability (Switzerland) 2022 Dec 1;14(24):16325.

[3] Tortajada C. Contributions of recycled wastewater to clean water and sanitation Sustainable Development Goals, 2020;22. URL: https://doi.org/10.1038/s41545-020-0069-3.

[4] Mizelle RM. A slow-moving disaster: The Jackson water crisis and the health effects of racism. New Engl J Med 2023;388(24):2212–4.

[5] Renwick DV, Heinrich A, Weisman R, Arvanaghi H, Rotert K. Potential public health impacts of deteriorating distribution system infrastructure. J Am Water Works Assoc 2019;111(2):42–53.

[6] Mississippi State Department of Health. Water supply. URL: https://msdh.ms.gov/page/30,0,76.html.

[7] United States Environmental Protection Agency. Summary of the Safe Drinking Water Act. EPA, 2023. URL: https://www.epa.gov/laws-regulations/summary-safe-drinking-water-act.

[8] Johnson Jr H. Challenges of an aging water system: The Jackson Water Crises: A research commentary. Mississippi Urban Research Center. Online J Rural Urban Res 2022;Spring:5-21.

[9] Kim M, De Vito R, Duarte F, Tieskens K, Luna M, Salazar-Miranda A, et al. Nature water: Boil water alerts and their impact on the unexcused absence rate in public schools in Jackson, Mississippi. Nature Water 2023;1:359–69. URL: https://doi.org/10.1038/s44221-023-00062-z.

[10] Rosner D. A lead poisoning crisis enters its second century. Health Aff 2016;35(5):756–9.

[11] Otts S, Janasie C. How safe is the water? An analysis of the lead contamination risks of public water supplies in the Mississippi Delta, 2017. URL: http://www.epa.gov/your-drinking-water/basic-.

[12] Zhang R, Wilson VL, Hou A, Meng G. Source of lead pollution, its influence on public health and the countermeasures. Int J Health Animal Sci Food Saf 2015;2(1):18-31.

[13] Debnath B, Singh W, Manna K. Sources and toxicological effects of lead on human health. Indian J Med Spec 2019;10(2):66.

[14] Masters RD, Coplan MJ. Water treatment with silicofluorides and lead toxicity. Int J Environ Stud 1999;56(4):435–49.
[15] Bacon SL, Mozee S. Lessons from Flint: A comparative study of water lead levels in Jackson, MS and 11 Southeastern Cities. Res Brief 2019;2(2):2-12.
[16] Wani AL, Ara A, Usmani JA. Lead toxicity: A review. Interdiscipl Toxicol 2015;8:55–64.
[17] Boskabady M, Marefati N, Farkhondeh T, Shakeri F, Farshbaf A, Boskabady MH. The effect of environmental lead exposure on human health and the contribution of inflammatory mechanisms. A review. Environ Int 2018;120:404–20.
[18] Kumar A, Kumar A, Cabral-Pinto M, Chaturvedi AK, Shabnam AA, Subrahmanyam G, et al. Lead toxicity: Health hazards, influence on food Chain, and sustainable remediation approaches. Int J Environ Res Public Health 2020;17(7):2179.
[19] Rees N, Fuller R, Narasimhan G, Solomon A, Design AB, Shangning V, et al. United Nations Environment Programme. New YorK: Nations Environment Programme, 2020.
[20] United States Centers for Disease Control and Prevention. Lead: Childhood blood lead surveillance data. Mississippi, 2023. URL: https://www.cdc.gov/nceh/lead/data/state/msdata.htm.
[21] United States Environmental Protection Agency. Lead laws and regulations. EPA, 2023. URL: https://www.epa.gov/lead/lead-laws-and-regulations.
[22] United States Environmental Protection Agency. Summary of the Toxic Substances Control Act. EPA, 2023. URL: https://www.epa.gov/laws-regulations/summary-toxic-substances-control-act.
[23] United States Environmental Protection Agency. Summary of the Clean Air Act. EPA, 2023. URL: https://www.epa.gov/laws-regulations/summary-clean-air-act.
[24] United States Environmental Protection Agency. Overview of the Safe Drinking Water Act. EPA, 2023. URL: https://www.epa.gov/sdwa/overview-safe-drinking-water-act.
[25] Collin MS, Venkatraman SK, Vijayakumar N, Kanimozhi V, Arbaaz SM, Stacey RGS, et al. Bioaccumulation of lead (Pb) and its effects on human: A review. J Hazardous Materials Adv 2022;7(2):100094.
[26] Giulioni C, Maurizi V, De Stefano V, Polisini G, Teoh JYC, Milanese G, et al. The influence of lead exposure on male semen parameters: A systematic review and meta-analysis. Reprod Toxicol 2023;118:108387.
[27] Senanayake J, Haji Rahman R, Safwat F, Riar S, Ampalloor G. Asymptomatic lead poisoning in a pediatric patient. Cureus 2023;15(2):e34940
[28] Chakraborty S, Ghosh A. A study of clinical presentations of chronic lead poisoning in adult. J Indian Med Assoc 2021;119(8):13-7.
[29] Schneider JS. Neurotoxicity and outcomes from developmental lead exposure: Persistent or permanent? Environ Health Perspect 2023;131(8):85002.
[30] United States Centers for Disease Control and Prevention. Testing children for lead poisoning, 2023. URL: https://www.cdc.gov/nceh/lead/prevention/testing-children-for-lead-poisoning.htm.

Chapter 6

Association of mercury exposure with allostatic load and cardiovascular disease risk

Hayley Howard, BS
and Emmanuel Obeng-Gyasi*, PhD, MPH

Department of Built Environment, North Carolina A&T State University,
Greensboro and Environmental Health and Disease Laboratory,
North Carolina A&T State University, Greensboro, North Carolina,
United States of America

Abstract

In this chapter we utilized data from NHANES 2017-2018 in order to explore the association of mercury exposure with allostatic load and cardiovascular disease risk among a representative sample of the United States non-institutionalized civilian population, involving 9,254 participants. The investigation provided critical insights including statistically significant relationships between mercury levels and diastolic blood pressure, total cholesterol and LDL Cholesterol in linear regression and triglycerides in logistic regression. These findings highlight the potential influence of environmental factors on cardiovascular health and the importance of integrating such factors into cardiovascular disease prevention and management strategies.

---

* *Correspondence:* Emmanuel Obeng-Gyasi, PhD, MPH, Department of Built Environment, North Carolina A&T State University, Greensboro and Environmental Health and Disease Laboratory, North Carolina A&T State University, Greensboro, North Carolina 27411, United States of America. Email: eobenggyasi@ncat.edu

In: Public Health: Understanding the Impact of Environmental Pollutants
Editors: Emmanuel Obeng-Gyasi and Joav Merrick
ISBN: 979-8-89530-579-9
© 2025 Nova Science Publishers, Inc.

Introduction

Globally, cardiovascular disease (CVD) stands as one of the primary contributors to mortality (1). CVD deaths have increased in numbers from 12.1 million recorded in 1990 to 18.6 million recorded in 2019. The numbers of people who die from CVD annually in the United States alone is more than 800,000 (2). According to the 2005 mortality rate data, it was found that approximately 2,400 Americans were dying from CVD each day (3). As the number of people affected by CVD rises, it's crucial to understand its primary causes. The most commonly linked risk factors to CVD include smoking, alcohol consumption, diabetes, and high cholesterol levels, which can affect blood vessels and contribute to cardiovascular issues (4). While these risk factors often stem from genetic predisposition or lifestyle choices, other influences, such as the environment, significantly contribute to CVD development (5-7). Emerging research reveals the impact of various environmental metals, including lead, aluminum, arsenic, cadmium, and mercury (8, 9). These metals often go unnoticed but play a role in CVD development (10).

Among heavy metals, mercury stands out as one of the most hazardous (11, 12). Mercury uniquely exists in gaseous, liquid, or solid states, with its elemental form, capable of global transportation when stable (10). Methylmercury, which is found to be the most hazardous form of mercury, is an organic compound that can be discovered as a pollutant in rivers, lakes, and oceans (13). Blood measurements can detect three forms of mercury: elemental, inorganic, and organic (14). Elemental and inorganic mercury have rapid half-lives in the blood of approximately 3 to 4 days, reflecting short-term exposure, primarily through inhalation or direct contact (15). Organic mercury, particularly methylmercury, has a longer half-life in the blood, estimated at approximately 50 days, indicating its bioaccumulation potential and dietary exposure through fish and shellfish consumption (16). The toxicity profiles of these mercury forms vary significantly. Elemental mercury primarily affects the central nervous system (CNS) and kidneys. Inorganic mercury compounds, having a higher solubility in water, can cause damage to the kidneys and gastrointestinal tract (17). Organic mercury compounds, especially methylmercury, are neurotoxic, readily crossing the blood-brain barrier and affecting the CNS, leading to neurological symptoms and cognitive impairments (17). The detection of mercury forms in blood is critical for assessing recent exposure (within the past day for elemental and inorganic mercury) and for the management of potential toxic effects, underscoring the importance of understanding their distinct toxicokinetic and toxicodynamic properties (18). There are various sources of where mercury can be found, it is naturally found in volcanoes and wildfires, human influence has also become a source of mercury exposure from coal burning and re-emission of formerly released mercury (19). According to the Environmental Protection Agency (EPA), the RfD for mercury is 0.1 microgram/kg each day, and any amount of mercury can cause health issues (10). Because of their ongoing physiological maturation, children exhibit increased susceptibility to mercury exposure (20). The accumulation of mercury in the human body adversely affects vital organs and systems, including the central nervous system, lungs, kidneys, skin, gastrointestinal tract, and cardiovascular system (21).

In a study involving males with myocardial infarction (MI) and using toenail mercury as a marker of exposure, researchers discovered a significant association between an increased risk of MI and elevated toenail mercury levels (10). Exposure to mercury triggers an upsurge in the generation of free radicals, reactive oxygen species (ROS), and superoxide anions, primarily induced by the Fenton reaction (11). This elevation of ROS levels and concurrent decline in antioxidant enzyme activity heighten susceptibility to cardiovascular diseases (11). Moreover, mercury exhibits its toxic effects by deactivating an extracellular antioxidative enzyme called paraoxonase (11). This enzyme assumes a critical role as an antioxidant for low-density lipoprotein (LDL), influencing the progression of atherosclerosis (22). Consequently, this disruption increases the risk of myocardial infarction, coronary heart disease, and carotid artery stenosis (13).

Allostatic load refers to the cumulative physiological toll exacted on the body due to prolonged stress responses (23). It encompasses the wear and tear on various physiological systems as they continuously adapt to stressors, striving to maintain stability and balance in response to environmental and psychological challenges (24). The paper's uses the allostatic load index, derived from an array of NHANES variables, including systolic and diastolic blood pressure, triglycerides, high-density lipoprotein cholesterol, total cholesterol, the inflammatory marker C-reactive protein, BMI, hemoglobin A1c, albumin, and creatinine clearance. Each of these variables is intricately linked to the concept of allostatic load (25), which represents the cumulative wear and tear on the body due to chronic exposure to stress. Systolic and diastolic blood pressure reflect cardiovascular stress (26), while triglycerides and cholesterol levels indicate metabolic and lipid balance (27). The C-reactive protein serves as a marker for systemic inflammation, often heightened in stress responses (28). Body mass index (BMI) is included as a measure of nutritional and metabolic status (29), hemoglobin A1c indicates long-term glucose control (30), and albumin and creatinine clearance provide insight into kidney function and protein metabolism (31). Collectively, these variables encompass the physiological domains affected by allostatic load, making them essential for a comprehensive assessment of an individual's physiological response to chronic stress and associated health risks.

Mercury exposure potentially contributes to an elevated allostatic load as indicated by its effect on markers which go into the allostatic load index (32). Mercury's relationship with the variables in the allostatic load index is multifaceted, reflecting its broad impact on various physiological systems. Exposure to mercury can lead to increased systolic and diastolic blood pressure by inducing oxidative stress and inflammation, damaging the endothelium of blood vessels, and altering autonomic nervous system function (33). It also disrupts lipid metabolism, leading to changes in triglycerides, high-density lipoprotein (HDL) cholesterol, and total cholesterol levels, as mercury's oxidative stress and inflammatory effects extend to the liver, affecting its function and lipid processing capabilities (13). In the context of inflammation, mercury exposure elevates C-reactive protein (CRP) levels, signifying systemic inflammation through the activation of immune responses and cytokine production (34).

Additionally, mercury can influence body mass index (BMI) by affecting metabolic rates, appetite regulation, and endocrine functions, particularly impacting the thyroid and adrenal glands (34,35). Its effect on glucose metabolism is evident in altered hemoglobin A1c levels, as mercury can impair pancreatic beta-cell function and insulin signaling pathways (36). Mercury's nephrotoxic properties are reflected in its impact on kidney function, notably decreasing creatinine clearance by accumulating in kidney tissues and causing cellular damage (37). Furthermore, mercury exposure can reduce albumin levels due to its detrimental effects on kidney and liver functions, essential for albumin synthesis and regulation (38). Collectively, these interactions highlight the pervasive influence of mercury on the physiological domains encompassed by the allostatic load index, underlining the critical need to consider environmental toxin exposure in assessing chronic stress and its health implications.

Mercury exposure in occupational and environmental settings, particularly in environments where mercury levels are elevated, introduces a significant health concern. Workers in industries such as mining, dental work, certain manufacturing processes, or waste management may face increased exposure to mercury through inhalation, skin contact, or ingestion of contaminated substances (39). The amalgamation of heightened mercury exposure and the confluence of stressors present in these work environments may significantly influence the body's stress response mechanisms. The physical and mental stressors, including job insecurity, and sometimes inadequate safety measures can collectively contribute to an increased burden on the body's adaptive systems (40). Mercury, known for its neurotoxic and oxidative stress-inducing properties, becomes an additional physiological stressor in this scenario. Exposure to elevated mercury levels prompts the release of stress hormones and triggers inflammatory responses in the body (41). This reaction is compounded by the pre-existing stressors present in the occupational environment, creating a synergistic effect that amplifies the body's response to stress.

Moreover, the social context of exposure to mercury in these environments cannot be overlooked as these social stressors add to the overall allostatic load experienced by individuals.

The combined effect of mercury exposure, physical and mental stressors in the workplace, and social stressors places a substantial strain on the body's regulatory systems. This chronic exposure to multiple stressors elevates the allostatic load, contributing to the wear and tear on various physiological systems. Over time, this increased load can lead to dysregulation in hormonal, cardiovascular, and immune systems, ultimately predisposing individuals to a higher risk of developing various health issues, including cardiovascular diseases, mental health disorders, and other stress-related conditions.

Our study

In this study, the hypothesis posits that exposure to mercury adversely affects allostatic load and cardiovascular disease risk by influencing indicators such as blood pressure, inflammation, and lipid profiles among the study participants. To investigate this hypothesis, the study aims to determine the impact of mercury exposure on cardiovascular and allostatic load markers, this study aims to assess the relationship between blood mercury levels (BMLs) and the levels of systolic blood pressure (SBP), diastolic blood pressure (DBP), C-reactive protein (CRP), triglycerides, total cholesterol, low-density lipoprotein (LDL) cholesterol, and high-density lipoprotein (HDL) cholesterol, as well as the overall allostatic load index, in a sample of United States adults.

We hypothesize that the potential pathways of disease from mercury exposure is via inflammation, leading to subsequent elevations in blood pressure and alterations in lipid metabolism. We also hypothesize that mercury acts on the HPA axis increasing the stress response.

Research design

The study utilized data from NHANES 2017–2018 to explore the association between mercury exposure, Allostatic load, and cardiovascular-related markers—SBP, DBP, CRP, total cholesterol, LDL cholesterol, HDL cholesterol, and triglycerides—within the general United States population. Data from the 2017–2018 datasets were processed using the NHANES web tutorial.

NHANES 2017–2018 survey, conducted by the CDC, encompassed a representative sample of the United States noninstitutionalized civilian population. This study involved 9,254 participants aged 38.43 years on average, representing approximately 320,842,721 people when factoring in NHANES survey design. Blood mercury was measured in 8,063 subjects, estimating around 293,304,132 people in the population. Additionally, blood pressure values were measured in 7,264 subjects, representing an estimated 276,076,185 people; CRP values in 7,800 subjects, representing approximately 285,617,337 people; triglycerides in 3,384 subjects, representing around 122,449,318 people. Total cholesterol was measured in 7,288 individuals, representing around 274,407,626 people, and HDL cholesterol data for the same number. LDL cholesterol values were measured in 3,358 individuals, representing approximately 121,263,507 people.

Biochemical markers were analyzed using standardized methods as indicated in the laboratory procedure manual (42). LDL cholesterol was calculated using Friedewald method while CRP was measured using an immunoturbidimetric assay where a specimen reacts with anti-CRP coated latex particles, causing turbidity proportional to CRP concentration, which is then quantified by light absorbance.

Metal assays in whole blood samples were conducted at the Division of Laboratory Sciences. Mercury levels are measured by diluting a whole blood specimen, which is then introduced into an Inductively Coupled Plasma Mass Spectrometer (ICP-MS), with the aid of a Dynamic Reaction Cell

(DRC) to reduce interference and increase ion signal, allowing precise quantification of total mercury content using assay method DLS 3016.8-06. All laboratory analyses were done at The Centers for Disease Control and Prevention (Division of Laboratory Sciences) (42).

Quantifying allostatic load

The study assessed allostatic load by considering specific markers including systolic blood pressure (SBP), diastolic blood pressure (DBP), triglycerides, high-density lipoprotein (HDL) cholesterol, total cholesterol, inflammatory marker C-reactive protein (CRP), and metabolic systems such as body mass index (BMI), hemoglobin A1C, albumin, and creatinine clearance.

The NHANES procedure for blood pressure measurement involved collecting a maximum of 3 readings for both systolic and diastolic BP using appropriate cuff sizes based on midarm circumference. Trained medical personnel adhered to a standard protocol, utilizing a Baumanometer true gravity mercury wall model at the MEC.

Triglycerides and HDL cholesterol levels were measured using the Roche modular P chemistry analyzer (Roche Diagnostics, Indianapolis, IN, USA). CRP levels were assessed via latex-enhanced nephelometry employing anti-CRP antibodies characterized by a hydrophilic shell and polystyrene core of CRP particles.

BMI was calculated as weight (kg) divided by the square of standing height (m^2), while glycohemoglobin was measured using the A1c G7 HPLC Glycohemoglobin Analyzer (Tosoh Medics, Inc., San Francisco, CA, USA). Urine creatinine was measured using the Roche/Hitachi Modular P Chemistry Analyzer (Roche Diagnostics, Indianapolis, IN, USA). Human urinary albumin was assessed using a non-competitive, double-antibody method, wherein an antibody was attached to human albumin, reacted with a urine specimen, and fluorescence of the resulting complex measured using a fluorometer (42). All laboratory analyses were done at The Centers for Disease Control and Prevention (Division of Laboratory Sciences) (42).

Operationalizing allostatic load

Drawing on previous research, an aggregate measure of physiological dysfunction encompassing cardiovascular (including SBP, DBP, triglycerides, HDL cholesterol, and total cholesterol), inflammatory (CRP), and metabolic indicators (BMI, hemoglobin A1c, albumin, and creatinine clearance) was constructed (23-25, 43-47). The biomarkers of allostatic load were segmented into four equal parts according to their frequency in the dataset. The highest risk category was designated for those within the uppermost quartile for most biomarkers, with the exception of albumin, creatinine clearance, and HDL cholesterol, where being in the lowest quartile indicated greater risk. A binary risk score was then attributed to each participant, with 1 indicating high risk and 0 indicating low risk across the biomarkers, resulting in a composite AL score with a maximum of 10. This study sought to use allostatic load as it has been previously used in similar studies. In conforming with the literature, an allostatic load score greater than or equal to 3 was considered high.

Statistical analysis

The data analytics techniques used in the study involved a combination of Spearman's correlation analysis, descriptive statistics, and linear regression analysis. Spearman's correlation was applied to assess the relationships among critical predictor variables highlighting both positive and negative correlations and their statistical significances. Descriptive statistics were utilized to summarize and describe the features of the dataset, providing insights into the distribution and central tendencies of the allostatic load (AL) markers and cardiovascular risk factors. Linear regression analysis examined the associations between mercury levels and various health variables, adjusted for age and BMI, identifying statistically significant predictors of mercury levels. In addition age and BMI adjusted, Binary logistic regression was performed with mercury as the binary outcome variable with values of 20 µg/L or higher set as high in the analysis. These techniques collectively facilitated a comprehensive analysis of the data, uncovering significant correlations and associations that inform the study's findings on the impact of mercury exposure on allostatic load and cardiovascular disease risk.

Data analysis and management

Data analysis and management adhered to NHANES analytical guidelines regarding survey design and weighting, and Stata SE 18 (StataCorp, College Station, TX, USA) and R (version 4.2.3; R Foundation for Statistical Computing, Vienna, Austria) was utilized for data management and analysis factoring in the survey design and weights into all analysis.

Our findings

Table 1 presents the demographic and health characteristics of participants categorized by allostatic load (AL) status. The table includes variables such as age at screening, body mass index (BMI), average systolic and diastolic blood pressure, HS C-Reactive Protein, total cholesterol, LDL-cholesterol, HDL-cholesterol, total blood mercury, and triglyceride levels. Values are reported separately for participants with high and low AL levels. The data indicate differences in these parameters between individuals with high and low AL, suggesting potential associations between allostatic load and various health markers.

Table 1. Clinical variables of interest in the study

Variable Name	High AL ≥3	Low AL <3	P value
Age in years at screening	38.16	40.78	0.009
Body Mass index (kg/m2)	27.98	25.04	< 0.0001
Average Systolic Blood Pressure	120.27	124.35	< 0.0001
Average Diastolic Blood Pressure	69.45	72.70	0.002
C-Reactive Protein (mg/L)	3.65	2.17	0.208
Total cholesterol (mg/dL)	184.89	172.16	< 0.0001
LDL-cholesterol (mg/dL)	111.84	98.86	< 0.0001
HDL-cholesterol (mg/dL)	52.86	58.91	< 0.0001
Total Blood mercury (ug/L)	1.15	1.08	0.559
Triglyceride (mg/dL)	120.83	71.96	< 0.0001

We performed spearman's correlation analysis of the critical predictor variables in the study (Figure 1). In figure, the red indicates that there is a positive correlation, and the blue indicates that there is a negative correlation. Analyzing the correlation plot and corresponding p-values for various biomedical measurements, we observe various degrees of relationships. CRP shows a moderate positive correlation with AL (0.43), implying they tend to increase together, but the p-value suggests this correlation is not statistically significant. AL is moderately correlated with triglycerides (0.48) and inversely with HDL-C (-0.37), yet these do not appear statistically significant either. Triglycerides and HDL-C present a notable negative correlation (-0.47), which is statistically significant, indicating an inverse relationship that holds true with statistical confidence.

LDL-C's correlation with HDL-C is also strongly negative (-0.47) and statistically significant, underscoring a robust inverse relationship. Additionally, LDL-C and total cholesterol exhibit a very strong positive correlation (0.92), with a significant p-value, reflecting a substantial direct association. However, the correlations between SBP and DBP with lipid measurements are generally weak and not statistically significant, though SBP and DBP themselves moderately correlate (0.49), hinting at a potential relationship between the two blood pressure measurements that is not supported by the p-value for significance.

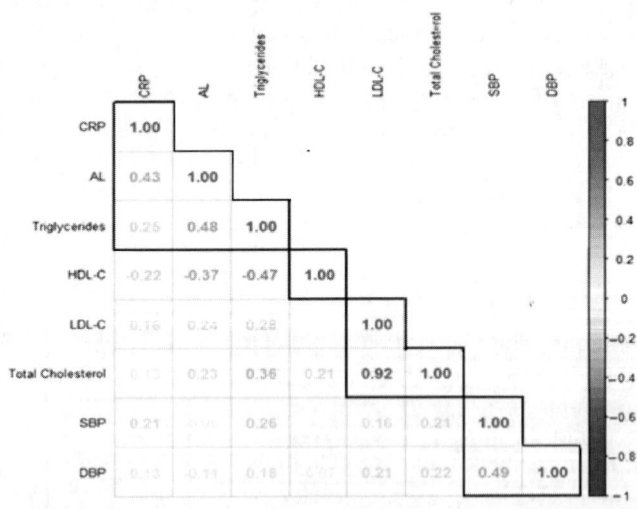

Figure 1. Correlation plot between predictor variables of interest.

Table 2 displays the results of a simple linear regression analysis examining the association between mercury levels and various health variables, adjusted for age. The table includes the variables CRP (C-Reactive Protein), SBP (Systolic Blood Pressure), DBP (Diastolic Blood Pressure), Triglycerides, Total Cholesterol, LDL Cholesterol, and HDL Cholesterol.

Table 2. Simple linear regression of relationship between mercury exposure and CVD variables

Variables	Mercury *adjusted Coefficient (95% CI)	p Value
AL	0.033(-0.015, 0.081)	0.160
CRP (mg/L)	-0.054(-0.304, 0.195)	0.651
SBP (mm Hg)	-0.188(-0.590, 0.214)	0.336
DBP (mm Hg)	0.312(0.101, 0.524)	0.007
Triglycerides (mg/dL)	0.224(-1.811, 2.260)	0.817
Total Cholesterol (mg/dL)	1.457(0.280, 2.633)	0.019
LDL Cholesterol (mg/dL)	1.209(0.101, 2.315)	0.034
HDL Cholesterol (mg/dL)	0.377(-0.097, 0.853)	0.111

*Adjusted for Age and BMI.

Table 3. Binary logistic regression of relationship between mercury exposure and CVD variables

Variables	Mercury *adjusted odds ratio (95% CI)	p Value
AL	1.20 (0.737, 1.960)	0.435
CRP (mg/L)	1.01(0.987, 1.04)	0.285
SBP (mm Hg)	1.01(0.972, 1.048)	0.614
DBP (mm Hg)	0.995(0.957, 1.033)	0.776
Triglycerides (mg/dL)	1.002(1.000, 1.003)	0.015
Total Cholesterol (mg/dL)	1.006(0.991, 1.021)	0.418
LDL Cholesterol (mg/dL)	1.010(0.999, 1.022)	0.069
HDL Cholesterol (mg/dL)	0.999(0.972, 1.028)	0.111

*Adjusted for Age and BMI.

The "mercury adjusted (95% CI)" column presents the estimated regression coefficients for each predictor variable, along with their corresponding 95% confidence intervals. The "p Value" column indicates the statistical significance of each predictor variable in predicting mercury levels.

The results suggest that DBP and Total Cholesterol are statistically significant predictors of mercury levels ($p < 0.05$), while SBP, CRP, Triglycerides, and HDL Cholesterol show no significant association with mercury levels ($p > 0.05$).

Binary logistic regression was performed with Mercury as the binary outcome variable with values of 20 μg/L or higher set as high in the analysis. The results can be found in Table 3. The results revealed that those with high triglycerides were significantly more likely to have mercury exposure ($p < 0.05$).

Discussion

This study investigated the association between mercury exposure, allostatic load (AL), and cardiovascular disease (CVD) risk. The results highlight several key findings regarding the interaction of these variables in the context of cardiovascular health.

Significant findings were observed in the strong negative correlation between triglycerides and HDL-C, as well as between HDL-C and LDL-C. The robust inverse relationship between these lipid profiles corroborates existing research suggesting that dyslipidemia is a key factor in the development of cardiovascular diseases (48). Moreover, the very strong positive correlation between LDL-C and total cholesterol, which was statistically significant, reinforces the central role of LDL-C in cardiovascular health and its potential utility as a primary target for intervention (49).

The inclusion of mercury as a variable in our study was premised on the hypothesis that mercury exposure could be associated with cardiovascular risk factors. The regression analysis indicated that mercury levels might be significantly associated with increases in DBP and total cholesterol and LDL Cholesterol, but no significant associations are observed with AL, CRP, SBP, triglycerides, and HDL Cholesterol. Logistic regression analysis on the other hand found significant relationships between mercury levels and triglycerides. Other works have found mercury to be associated with both systolic blood pressure in the Brazilian Amazon (50), and among Nunavik Inuit adults (51), a study among US individuals aged 16-49 years found no association between mercury and blood pressure in multivariate models (52). In a study of dental professionals by Xu and colleagues no significant associations between mercury and lipid levels or blood pressure was found (53). On the other hand in a study of Korean adults by Kang and colleagues significant associations were found between mercury and dyslipidemia (54). These findings underscore the need for further investigation into the potential mechanisms by which mercury could influence lipid metabolism. While the precise pathways remain unclear, one possibility is that mercury exposure contributes to oxidative stress and inflammation, thereby affecting lipid profiles and contributing to cardiovascular risk (33).

This study posited that the stress pathway, specifically the physiological responses to chronic stress represented by allostatic load, might mediate the relationship between mercury exposure and cardiovascular disease risk (23). However, findings suggest that this pathway may not play a central role in linking mercury exposure to CVD risk. Several factors could contribute to the diminished mediating effect of AL in this context:

Firstly, mercury's impact on cardiovascular health may not follow a linear trajectory; instead, it could exhibit threshold effects where its deleterious impacts only become manifest beyond certain exposure levels (55,56). Such dynamics might not align neatly with the incremental changes captured by allostatic load markers, thus obscuring potential mediation effects.

It may also speak to the direct toxicological effects of mercury. Mercury has known neurotoxic and oxidative stress-inducing properties, which can directly affect cardiovascular health independent of stress pathways (57). Mercury's ability to induce oxidative stress, inflammation, and disrupt lipid metabolism directly interferes with cardiovascular functions (58). These direct actions may not necessitate the intermediation of allostatic load for their impact on cardiovascular risk to be evident.

Additionally, there is complexity of allostatic load as a mediator. Allostatic load encapsulates a broad spectrum of physiological responses to stress, encompassing cardiovascular, metabolic, and immune systems (25, 59). This complexity might dilute the specific pathways through which mercury exerts its influence, making it challenging to pinpoint AL as a critical mediator (60). Furthermore, the components of AL might not be sensitive or specific enough to capture the nuanced changes induced by mercury exposure (61).

There may also exist interindividual variability in response to mercury exposure (62). Individual differences in genetic susceptibility, antioxidant capacity, and previous exposure to stressors can influence how mercury exposure impacts health. These individual variations might modulate the relationship between mercury and cardiovascular risk in ways that are not adequately accounted for by measures of allostatic load.

Finally, temporal aspects of mercury exposure and allostatic load accumulation may be a factor (63). The timing and duration of mercury exposure relative to the accumulation of allostatic load could also play a role. Long-term, low-level exposure to mercury might have cumulative effects that are not immediately reflected in allostatic load measurements but still contribute to cardiovascular risk over time.

The implications of the findings of our study are multifaceted. They suggest that while traditional cardiovascular risk factors such as diet remain critical, environmental exposures may also play a role in cardiovascular health. This underscores the importance of considering environmental factors in the prevention and management of cardiovascular diseases (64).

However, this study is not without limitations. The cross-sectional nature of the study design precludes us from making causal inferences. Moreover, the reliance on self-reported data for some variables could introduce reporting bias. Future longitudinal studies are necessary to establish temporal relationships and causality between mercury exposure, AL, and CVD risk.

Conclusion

In conclusion, the study sheds light on the complex relationship between mercury exposure, allostatic load, and cardiovascular disease risk. Although the expected significant correlations between allostatic load and various markers like CRP was not observed, possibly due to unaccounted confounding factors or an inadequate sample size, there were significant findings. Notably, the research highlighted a statistically significant association between mercury and diastolic blood pressure, total cholesterol and LDL cholesterol in linear regression, while logistic regression showed significant associations with triglycerides suggesting a potential impact of mercury on lipid metabolism and cardiovascular health. These findings underscore the importance of considering environmental factors in the assessment of cardiovascular disease risk, alongside traditional risk factors, and point to the need for further research to unravel the mechanisms by which mercury influences health outcomes.

Acknowledgments

Conceptualization, E.O.-G.; methodology, E.O.-G; formal analysis, H.H., E.O.-G..; investigation, H.H., E.O.-G.; resources, E.O.-G.; data curation, E.O.-G.; writing—original draft preparation, H.H., and E.O.-G.; writing—review and editing, H.H., E.O.-G; supervision, E.O.-G.; project administration, E.O.-G.; funding acquisition, E.O.-G. All authors have read and agreed to the published version of the manuscript.

Funding: Research reported in this publication was supported by the National Institute of General Medical Sciences of the National Institutes of

Health under Award Number R16GM149473. The content is solely the responsibility of the authors and does not necessarily represent the official views of the National Institutes of Health.

References

[1] Kirla H, Henry DJ, Jansen S, Thompson PL, Hamzah J. Use of silica nanoparticles for drug delivery in cardiovascular disease. Clin Ther 2023;45(11):1060-8.
[2] Han SN. Vegetarian diet for cardiovascular disease risk reduction: Cons J Lipid Atheroscler 2023;12(3):323-8.
[3] Jennrich P. The influence of arsenic, lead, and mercury on the development of cardiovascular diseases. ISRN Hypertension 2013;2013:1-15.
[4] Chen Z, Tao T, Huang G, Tong X, Li Q, Su G. Analysis of the association between serum antiaging humoral factor klotho and cardiovascular disease potential risk factor apolipoprotein B in general population. Medicine (Baltimore) 2023;102(25):e34056.
[5] Bhatnagar A. Environmental determinants of cardiovascular disease. Circ Res 2017;121(2):162-80.
[6] Sing CF, Stengård JH, Kardia SL. Genes, environment, and cardiovascular disease. Arterioscler Thromb Vasc Biol 2003;23(7):1190-6.
[7] Rankinen T, Sarzynski MA, Ghosh S, Bouchard C. Are there genetic paths common to obesity, cardiovascular disease outcomes, and cardiovascular risk factors? Circ Res 2015;116(5):909-22.
[8] Liu Z, He C, Chen M, Yang S, Li J, Lin Y, et al. The effects of lead and aluminum exposure on congenital heart disease and the mechanism of oxidative stress. Reprod Toxicol 2018;81:93-8.
[9] Solenkova NV, Newman JD, Berger JS, Thurston G, Hochman JS, Lamas GA. Metal pollutants and cardiovascular disease: mechanisms and consequences of exposure. Am Heart J 2014;168(6):812-22.
[10] Houston MC. The role of mercury in cardiovascular disease. J Cardiovasc Dis Diagn. 2014;2:1-8.
[11] Balali-Mood M, Sadeghi M. Toxic mechanisms of five heavy metals: mercury, lead, chromium, cadmium, and arsenic. Front Pharmacol 2021;12:643972.
[12] Jyothi NR, Farook NAM. Mercury toxicity in public health. In: Nduka JK Rashed MN, eds. Heavy metal toxicity in public health. London: IntechOpen, 2020:1-12.
[13] Genchi G, Sinicropi MS, Carocci A, Lauria G, Catalano A. Mercury exposure and heart diseases. Int J Environ Res Public Health 2017;14(1):74.
[14] Park J-D, Zheng W. Human exposure and health effects of inorganic and elemental mercury. J Prev Med Public Health 2012;45(6):344.
[15] Aylward LL, Kirman CR, Schoeny R, Portier CJ, Hays SM. Evaluation of biomonitoring data from the CDC National Exposure Report in a risk assessment context: perspectives across chemicals. Environ Health Perspect 2013;121(3):287-94.

[16] Risher JF, Murray HE, Prince GR. Organic mercury compounds: human exposure and its relevance to public health. Toxicol Ind Health 2002;18(3):109-60.
[17] Zulaikhah ST, Wahyuwibowo J, Pratama AA. Mercury and its effect on human health: A review of the literature. Int J Public Health Sci 2020;9(2):103-14.
[18] Okpala COR, Sardo G, Vitale S, Bono G, Arukwe A. Hazardous properties and toxicological update of mercury: From fish food to human health safety perspective. Crit Rev Food Sci Nutr 2018;58(12):1986-2001.
[19] Gworek B, Dmuchowski W, Baczewska-Dąbrowska AH. Mercury in the terrestrial environment: A review. Environ Sci Europe 2020;32(1):128.
[20] Bose-O'Reilly S, McCarty KM, Steckling N, Lettmeier B. Mercury exposure and children's health. Curr Probl Pediatr Adolesc Health Care 2010;40(8):186-215.
[21] Kampalath RA, Jay JA. Sources of mercury exposure to children in low- and middle-income countries. J Health Pollut 2015;5(8):33-51.
[22] Ahmad S, Mahmood R. Mercury chloride toxicity in human erythrocytes: enhanced generation of ROS and RNS, hemoglobin oxidation, impaired antioxidant power, and inhibition of plasma membrane redox system. Environ Sci Pollut Res 2019;26:5645-57.
[23] McEwen BS. Stress, adaptation, and disease: Allostasis and allostatic load. Ann NY Acad Sci 1998;840(1):33-44.
[24] McEwen BS. Protection and damage from acute and chronic stress: allostasis and allostatic overload and relevance to the pathophysiology of psychiatric disorders. Ann NY Acad Sci 2004;1032(1):1-7.
[25] McEwen BS, Gianaros PJ. Central role of the brain in stress and adaptation: links to socioeconomic status, health, and disease. Ann NY Acad Sci 2010;1186(1):190-222.
[26] Matthews KA, Katholi CR, McCreath H, Whooley MA, Williams DR, Zhu S, et al. Blood pressure reactivity to psychological stress predicts hypertension in the CARDIA study. Circulation 2004;110(1):74-8.
[27] Laufs U, Parhofer KG, Ginsberg HN, Hegele RA. Clinical review on triglycerides. Eur Heart J 2020;41(1):99-109.
[28] Marsland AL, Walsh C, Lockwood K, John-Henderson NA. The effects of acute psychological stress on circulating and stimulated inflammatory markers: a systematic review and meta-analysis. Brain Behav Immunity 2017;64:208-19.
[29] Weisell RC. Body mass index as an indicator of obesity. Asia Pac J Clin Nutr 2002;11:S681-S4.
[30] Vigersky RA, McMahon C. The relationship of hemoglobin A1C to time-in-range in patients with diabetes. Diabetes Technol Ther 2019;21(2):81-5.
[31] Lopez-Giacoman S, Madero M. Biomarkers in chronic kidney disease, from kidney function to kidney damage. World J Nephrol 2015;4(1):57.
[32] Virtanen JK, Rissanen TH, Voutilainen S, Tuomainen T-P. Mercury as a risk factor for cardiovascular diseases. J Nutr Biochem 2007;18(2):75-85.
[33] Houston MC. Role of mercury toxicity in hypertension, cardiovascular disease, and stroke. J Clin Hypertension 2011;13(8):621-7.
[34] Kim K, Park H. Association of mercury exposure with the serum high-sensitivity C-reactive protein level in Korean adults. Front Public Health 2023;11:1062741.

[35] Wada H, Cristol DA, McNabb FA, Hopkins WA. Suppressed adrenocortical responses and thyroid hormone levels in birds near a mercury-contaminated river. Environ Sci Technol 2009;43(15):6031-8.

[36] Roy C, Tremblay P-Y, Ayotte P. Is mercury exposure causing diabetes, metabolic syndrome and insulin resistance? A systematic review of the literature. Environ Res 2017;156:747-60.

[37] Sällsten G, Barregård L, Schütz A. Clearance half-life of mercury in urine after the cessation of long term occupational exposure: influence of a chelating agent (DMPS) on excretion of mercury in urine. Occup Environ Med 1994;51(5):337-42.

[38] Song S, Li Y, Liu QS, Wang H, Li P, Shi J, et al. Interaction of mercury ion (Hg2+) with blood and cytotoxicity attenuation by serum albumin binding. J Hazard Mater 2021;412:125158.

[39] Ratcliffe HE, Swanson GM, Fischer LJ. Human exposure to mercury: a critical assessment of the evidence of adverse health effects. J Toxicol Environ Health 1996;49(3):221-70.

[40] De Castro A, Voss JG, Ruppin A, Dominguez CF, Seixas NS. Stressors among Latino day laborers: A pilot study examining allostatic load. AAOHN J 2010;58(5):185-96.

[41] Tan SW, Meiller JC, Mahaffey KR. The endocrine effects of mercury in humans and wildlife. Crit Rev Toxicol 2009;39(3):228-69.

[42] Centers for Disease Control and Prevention. Laboratory procedure manual. URL: https://wwwn.cdc.gov/nchs/data/nhanes/2015-2016/labmethods/PFAS_I_MET.pdf.

[43] McEwen BS. Mood disorders and allostatic load. Biol Psychiatry 2003;54(3):200-7.

[44] Obeng-Gyasi E, Obeng-Gyasi B. Chronic stress and cardiovascular disease among individuals exposed to lead: A pilot study. Diseases 2020;8(1):7.

[45] Obeng-Gyasi E, Ferguson AC, Stamatakis KA, Province MA. Combined effect of lead exposure and allostatic load on cardiovascular disease mortality—a preliminary study. Int J Environ Res Public Health 2021;18(13):6879.

[46] Hill M, Obeng-Gyasi E. The association of cytomegalovirus IgM and allostatic load. Diseases 2022;10(4):70.

[47] Boafo YS, Mostafa S, Obeng-Gyasi E. Association of combined metals and PFAS with cardiovascular disease risk. Toxics 2023;11(12):979.

[48] Hedayatnia M, Asadi Z, Zare-Feyzabadi R, Yaghooti-Khorasani M, Ghazizadeh H, Ghaffarian-Zirak R, et al. Dyslipidemia and cardiovascular disease risk among the MASHAD study population. Lipids Health Dis 2020;19:1-11.

[49] Barter P, Gotto AM, LaRosa JC, Maroni J, Szarek M, Grundy SM, et al. HDL cholesterol, very low levels of LDL cholesterol, and cardiovascular events. N Engl J Med 2007;357(13):1301-10.

[50] Fillion M, Mergler D, Passos CJS, Larribe F, Lemire M, Guimarães JRD. A preliminary study of mercury exposure and blood pressure in the Brazilian Amazon. Environ Health 2006;5:1-9.

[51] Valera B, Dewailly E, Poirier P. Environmental mercury exposure and blood pressure among Nunavik Inuit adults. Hypertension 2009;54(5):981-6.

[52] Vupputuri S, Longnecker MP, Daniels JL, Guo X, Sandler DP. Blood mercury level and blood pressure among US women: results from the National Health and Nutrition Examination Survey 1999–2000. Environ Res 2005;97(2):195-200.
[53] Xu W, Park SK, Gruninger SE, Charles S, Franzblau A, Basu N, et al. Associations between mercury exposure with blood pressure and lipid levels: A cross-sectional study of dental professionals. Environ Res 2023;220:115229.
[54] Kang P, Shin HY, Kim KY. Association between dyslipidemia and mercury exposure in adults. Int J Environ Res Public Health 2021;18(2):775.
[55] Ye B-J, Kim B-G, Jeon M-J, Kim S-Y, Kim H-C, Jang T-W, et al. Evaluation of mercury exposure level, clinical diagnosis and treatment for mercury intoxication. Ann Occup Environ Med 2016;28(1):1-8.
[56] Hu XF, Singh K, Chan HM. Mercury exposure, blood pressure, and hypertension: A systematic review and dose–response meta-analysis. Environ Health Perspect 2018;126(07):076002.
[57] Gokoel AR, Zijlmans WC, Covert HH, Abdoel Wahid F, Shankar A, MacDonald-Ottevanger MS, et al. Influence of prenatal exposure to mercury, perceived stress, and depression on birth outcomes in Suriname: results from the MeKiTamara study. Int J Environ Res Public Health 2020;17(12):4444.
[58] Zhao Y, Zhou C, Guo X, Hu G, Li G, Zhuang Y, et al. Exposed to mercury-induced oxidative stress, changes of intestinal microflora, and association between them in mice. Biol Trace Elem Res 2021;199:1900-7.
[59] Bashir T, Obeng-Gyasi E. Combined effects of multiple per-and polyfluoroalkyl substances exposure on allostatic load using Bayesian Kernel Machine Regression. Int J Environ Res Public Health 2023;20(10):5808.
[60] Bashir T, Obeng-Gyasi E. The association between multiple per-and polyfluoroalkyl substances' serum levels and allostatic load. Int J Environ Res Public Health 2022;19(9):5455.
[61] Carbone JT, Clift J, Alexander N. Measuring allostatic load: Approaches and limitations to algorithm creation. J Psychosom Res 2022;163:111050.
[62] Berglund M, Lind B, Björnberg KA, Palm B, Einarsson Ö, Vahter M. Inter-individual variations of human mercury exposure biomarkers: A cross-sectional assessment. Environ Health 2005;4:1-11.
[63] Gustafsson PE, Janlert U, Theorell T, Westerlund H, Hammarström A. Socioeconomic status over the life course and allostatic load in adulthood: Results from the Northern Swedish Cohort. J Epidemiol Community Health 2011;65(11):986-92.
[64] Cosselman KE, Navas-Acien A, Kaufman JD. Environmental factors in cardiovascular disease. Nat Rev Cardiol 2015;12(11):627-42.

Chapter 7

Association of total arsenic exposure with allostatic load and cardiovascular disease risk

Elon Barbee, BS
and Emmanuel Obeng-Gyasi*, PhD, MPH
Department of Built Environment, North Carolina A&T State University,
Greensboro and Environmental Health and Disease Laboratory,
North Carolina A&T State University, Greensboro, North Carolina,
United States of America

Abstract

In this chapter we investigated the relationship between arsenic exposure (as measured in urine) and both allostatic load and cardiovascular disease (CVD) risk markers within a representative group of participants from the United States non-institutionalized civilian population. The results revealed individuals with high arsenic levels were significantly older than those with lower arsenic levels. Other findings indicated no significant associations between cardiovascular variables by degree of arsenic exposure as measured by total urinary arsenic. These results underscore the need to assess numerous biomarkers when examining the potential health implications of exposure to arsenic as markers of longer-term Arsenic exposure or consideration of specificity of arsenic species may have yielded different results.

---

* **Correspondence:** Emmanuel Obeng-Gyasi, PhD, MPH, Department of Built Environment, North Carolina A&T State University, Greensboro and Environmental Health and Disease Laboratory, North Carolina A&T State University, Greensboro, North Carolina 27411, United States of America. Email: eobenggyasi@ncat.edu

In: Public Health: Understanding the Impact of Environmental Pollutants
Editors: Emmanuel Obeng-Gyasi and Joav Merrick
ISBN: 979-8-89530-579-9
© 2025 Nova Science Publishers, Inc.

Introduction

Cardiovascular disease (CVD) is the primary cause of death globally and a significant contributor to disability. It continues to be a major health concern in the United States, significantly impacting health care costs (1). As the population grows, the global cardiovascular disease burden continues to increase, particularly among older adults; nevertheless, better cardiovascular care and advances in medicine have significantly reshaped the epidemiology of CVD and have created new patient profiles over time resulting in better care for even the most ill patients (2).

Conventional risk factors for CVD

Several well-established conventional risk factors contribute to the development of CVD. Among these are hypertension, hypercholesterolemia, diabetes mellitus, and smoking, which have been identified as significant contributors to the disease's onset and progression (3) A large-scale study involving approximately 500,000 patients' medical records provided insightful data on the prevalence of these risk factors among individuals newly diagnosed with CVD. The findings revealed that 40.7% of these patients had hypertension, 41.7% suffered from hypercholesterolemia, 16.5% were diagnosed with diabetes mellitus, and 28.2% had been or were current smokers (4). These statistics highlight the critical need for targeted interventions and lifestyle modifications to mitigate these risk factors, emphasizing the importance of regular screening and preventive measures in the fight against cardiovascular disease.

Emerging research on environmental factors in CVD development

Emerging research has increasingly highlighted the significance of environmental factors in the development of CVD, pointing towards a complex interplay between lifestyle, socio-economic status (SES), and environmental exposures (5).

A study by Teshale and colleagues (6) found that Environmental attributes such as proximity to a major road, reduced access to food stores, lack of recreational areas, increased access to fast-food restaurants, high distance from healthcare care facilities, and high traffic density were associated with a higher risk of coronary heart disease, myocardial infarction, heart failure, stroke, and angina in addition, lower neighborhood SES was associated with a higher risk of composite CVD, stroke, coronary heart disease, heart failure, and composite CVD mortality (6).

In addition, toxic environmental exposures, such as lead, arsenic, cadmium, and mercury, could be intricately linked to the pathogenesis of CVD. These metals, often pervasive in areas with high industrial activities or poor waste management practices, can induce oxidative stress, inflammation, and endothelial dysfunction, further exacerbating cardiovascular risk (7-9).

Role of arsenic exposure

Arsenic, a regulated hazardous material, constitutes a significant environmental, agricultural, and health challenge, representing a critical risk factor for human exposure. Naturally occurring in the Earth's crust, arsenic emanates from geogenic sources, with its distribution being highly variable. It averages in concentration across various geological formations and is found in over 200 mineral forms, with arsenopyrite being the most prevalent. Anthropogenic activities, notably mining, metal smelting, and the combustion of fossil fuels, substantially augment the environmental burden of arsenic, leading to its dispersion in the air, water, and soil.

Industrially, arsenic contamination is primarily attributed to high-temperature processes, such as those encountered in coal-fired power stations and the incineration of vegetation, alongside emissions from volcanic activities. The atmospheric presence of arsenic, particularly in industrial zones, is predominantly linked to the release of airborne particulates during the smelting of ores and the combustion of coal, highlighting air as a significant vector for arsenic exposure. This multifaceted presence of arsenic underscores the complex pathways through which it can affect environmental and human health, necessitating comprehensive strategies for monitoring, regulation, and mitigation to address its pervasive impact (10).

Accumulation of arsenic in the human body

Inorganic arsenic is recognized as a potent human carcinogen implicated in the etiology of various cancers, including those of the skin, lung, and bladder

(11). Moreover, a growing body of literature has highlighted its significant correlations with liver, prostate, and kidney malignancies (12). Beyond its carcinogenic properties, recent investigative efforts have proposed associations between inorganic arsenic exposure and a range of non-cancerous health outcomes, such as diabetes, neurological impairments, cardiac disorders, and adverse effects on reproductive health (13, 14). However, these findings necessitate further empirical validation to solidify the connections.

A notable study conducted by Lee et al. (15) using animal models delves into the impact of arsenic on thrombocytes, which are critical in the pathogenesis of cardiovascular diseases. Their research elucidates that trivalent arsenite, in the presence of thrombin, significantly enhances the agglutination of thrombocytes—a process integral to clot formation and, by extension, cardiovascular pathologies. Furthermore, Lee and colleagues postulate that chronic exposure to arsenic-laden drinking water exacerbates thrombocyte agglutination, potentially elevating the risk for cardiovascular diseases. This hypothesis underscores the intricate relationship between arsenic exposure and cardiovascular health, suggesting a mechanistic pathway through which arsenic contributes to cardiovascular disease risk (15).

Cardiovascular system as a primary target

A substantial body of research has focused on elucidating the impact of arsenic exposure on cardiovascular risk factors, revealing critical insights into its detrimental effects on cardiovascular health (16). These studies collectively demonstrate that both high and moderately-high levels of arsenic exposure can induce oxidative stress, inflammation, and endothelial dysfunction within the vasculature. These pathological states are closely linked to an elevated risk of developing cardiovascular diseases (CVD), underscoring the toxicological mechanisms through which arsenic exerts its harmful cardiovascular effects (17).

Further investigations, particularly those involving participants from the United States exposed to moderate levels of arsenic, have identified a robust positive correlation between arsenic exposure—as measured by urinary arsenic levels—and the incidence of CVD, coronary heart disease, and stroke mortality (18). Such findings not only reinforce the association between arsenic exposure and cardiovascular risk but also suggest the cardiovascular system as a primary target of arsenic's toxic effects.

The oxidative stress induced by arsenic exposure is characterized by an imbalance between the production of reactive oxygen species (ROS) and the body's ability to detoxify these reactive intermediates or repair the resulting damage (19). This oxidative stress, in turn, contributes to the initiation and progression of atherosclerosis by damaging endothelial cells lining the blood vessels, a key event in the pathogenesis of cardiovascular diseases. Concurrently, arsenic-induced inflammation acts as a pivotal mechanism, further exacerbating vascular damage and promoting the development of atherosclerotic plaques. Moreover, the impairment of endothelial function—a critical regulator of vascular tone and homeostasis—by arsenic exposure highlights a direct pathway through which arsenic contributes to cardiovascular morbidity (20).

The consistent findings across these studies highlight the grave public health implications of arsenic exposure and call for urgent strategies to mitigate arsenic contamination in the environment. Additionally, these insights pave the way for further research to explore potential interventions that could ameliorate the cardiovascular effects of arsenic exposure, thereby reducing the burden of cardiovascular diseases in affected populations.

Allostatic load and its interplay with arsenic exposure and CVD

Arsenic exposure in the context of chronic stress may exacerbate CVD and related conditions. Allostatic load—a measure of the cumulative burden of chronic stress and life events on the body—has been increasingly recognized as pivotal factor in CVD risk. Allostatic load encapsulates the physiological consequences of chronic exposure to fluctuating or heightened neural or neuroendocrine response that results from repeated or prolonged environmental challenges (21, 22). When individuals are exposed to environmental contaminants such as arsenic, either through contaminated water, food, or occupational settings, they may trigger a cascade of biological responses to maintain homeostasis (23). However, this adaptive process can become maladaptive when the exposure is chronic, leading to oxidative stress, inflammation, and endothelial dysfunction, all of which are markers of increased allostatic load. This enhanced allostatic load, in turn, may exacerbate the risk of developing CVD by impairing the body's ability to regulate blood pressure, lipid metabolism, and glucose levels, and by promoting atherogenesis (24). The relationship between arsenic exposure, allostatic load, and cardiovascular disease risk underscores the intricate interplay between environmental toxins and the body's stress response mechanisms, highlighting the need for holistic approaches to manage environmental health risks and prevent CVD (25).

Purpose and organization of the paper

Our paper aims to investigate and elucidate the complex relationship between arsenic exposure, its contribution to allostatic load, and the risk of developing cardiovascular diseases (CVD). Given the widespread occurrence of arsenic in the environment and its recognized status as a potent contaminant with far-reaching health impacts, this study aims to deepen the understanding of how exposure to arsenic can exacerbate physiological stress mechanisms, thereby increasing the allostatic load and elevating the risk for CVD. By exploring these associations, we seek to fill critical gaps in the current scientific literature, providing a clearer picture of the mechanistic pathways through which arsenic influences cardiovascular health. Ultimately, the findings of this paper are intended to inform public health strategies, policy-making, and clinical practices to mitigate the CVD risks associated with arsenic exposure, thereby contributing to the broader efforts to reduce the global burden of cardiovascular diseases.

Our study

In this study, the hypothesis suggests that exposure to total arsenic (organic plus inorganic) adversely affects allostatic load and cardiovascular disease risk by impacting the study participants' blood pressure, inflammation, and lipid profiles. To explore this hypothesis, the study aims to determine the impact of arsenic exposure on cardiovascular and allostatic load markers. Specifically, this study seeks to assess the relationship between total arsenic levels (TALs) in blood and the levels of systolic blood pressure (SBP), diastolic blood pressure (DBP), C-reactive protein (CRP), triglycerides, total cholesterol, low-density lipoprotein (LDL) cholesterol, and high-density lipoprotein (HDL) cholesterol, as well as the overall allostatic load index, in a sample of United States adults.

We hypothesize that the potential pathways of disease from arsenic exposure are through inflammation, which may lead to subsequent elevations in blood pressure and alterations in lipid metabolism. We also hypothesize that arsenic affects the hypothalamic-pituitary-adrenal (HPA) axis, increasing the stress response.

Research design

The study utilized data from NHANES 2017–2018 to explore the association between total arsenic exposure, allostatic load, and cardiovascular-related markers—SBP, DBP, CRP, total cholesterol, LDL cholesterol, HDL cholesterol, and triglycerides—within the general United States population. The 2017–2018 data were processed using the NHANES web tutorial.

The NHANES 2017–2018 survey, conducted by the CDC, encompassed a representative sample of the United States noninstitutionalized civilian population. This study involved 9,254 participants aged 38.43 years on average. Blood total arsenic levels were measured in a subset of these participants, along with measurements of blood pressure, CRP levels, triglycerides, total cholesterol, HDL cholesterol, and LDL cholesterol.

Biochemical markers were analyzed using standardized methods described in the laboratory procedure manual. LDL cholesterol levels were calculated using the Friedewald method, and CRP levels were measured with an immunoturbidimetric assay. Details of these processes and the metal assays, including the measurement of arsenic levels via Inductively Coupled Plasma Mass Spectrometry (ICP-MS), can be found in the manual. All analyses were conducted at the Centers for Disease Control and Prevention, Division of Laboratory Sciences (26).

Quantifying allostatic load

The research measured allostatic load through various indicators such as systolic and diastolic blood pressure (SBP and DBP), triglycerides, HDL cholesterol, total cholesterol, the inflammatory biomarker C-reactive protein (CRP), and metabolic markers like body mass index (BMI), hemoglobin A1C, albumin, and creatinine clearance.

The NHANES guidelines were followed for blood pressure measurements, which involve taking up to three readings using cuffs sized according to the participant's midarm circumference. These measurements were conducted by trained health professionals.

The Roche modular P chemistry analyzer determined levels of triglyceride and HDL cholesterol. CRP was quantified through a process of latex-enhanced nephelometry that utilizes anti-CRP antibodies.

BMI was determined by dividing the weight in kilograms by the square of height in meters. Hemoglobin A1C levels were analyzed using the Tosoh Medics A1c G7 HPLC Glycohemoglobin Analyzer. Creatinine in urine was assessed with the Roche/Hitachi Modular P Chemistry Analyzer. Albumin in human urine was measured through a dual-antibody technique where antibodies specific to human albumin were used, and the fluorescence of the formed complex was measured with a fluorometer (26).

Operationalizing allostatic load

Building on earlier studies, a composite index was developed to gauge physiological dysfunction. This index includes cardiovascular measures such as systolic and diastolic blood pressure, triglycerides, HDL cholesterol, and total cholesterol, along with inflammatory and metabolic markers including C-reactive protein (CRP), body mass index (BMI), hemoglobin A1c, albumin, and creatinine clearance (21-24,27-30). The allostatic load biomarkers in the study were divided into quartiles based on their distribution within the dataset. For most biomarkers, participants in the highest quartile were categorized as the highest-risk group. However, being in the lowest quartile was associated with increased risk for albumin, creatinine clearance, and HDL cholesterol. Participants were then assigned a binary risk score—1 for high risk and 0 for low risk—for each biomarker, culminating in an overall allostatic load (AL) score out of a possible 10. This study used the allostatic load metric, commonly applied in prior research. Following established literature, an allostatic load score of 3 or higher was classified as high.

Statistical analysis

The data analytics techniques used in the study involved a combination of Spearman's correlation analysis, descriptive statistics, and linear regression analysis. Spearman's correlation was applied to assess the relationships among critical predictor variables, highlighting both positive and negative correlations and their statistical significance. Descriptive statistics were utilized to summarize and describe the features of the dataset, providing insights into the distribution and central tendencies of the allostatic load (AL) markers and cardiovascular risk factors. Linear regression analysis examined the associations between arsenic levels and various health variables, adjusted for age initially and then further adjusted for urinary creatinine, gender, BMI, Alcohol, and Ethnicity if significance was found. This helped identify statistically significant predictors of arsenic levels. In addition, age and BMI adjusted.

Data analysis and management

Data analysis and management adhered to NHANES analytical guidelines regarding survey design and weighting, and Stata SE 18 (StataCorp, College Station, TX, USA) and R (version 4.2.3; R Foundation for Statistical Computing, Vienna, Austria) were utilized for data management and analysis factoring in the survey design and weights into all analysis.

Our findings

Table 1 presents a comparative analysis of various clinical variables based on urinary arsenic levels in participants. The variables are divided into two categories: individuals with high urinary arsenic levels (greater than 50 mcg/L) and those with low levels (50 mcg/L or less). The analysis reveals that the average age at screening is significantly higher in the high arsenic group at 52.08 years, compared to 43.57 years in the low arsenic group, with a p-value of 0.001, indicating statistical significance. While differences in body mass index (BMI) and blood pressure measurements (both systolic and diastolic) are observed between the two groups, these are not statistically significant, as the p-values are above 0.05. The lipid profiles, which include total cholesterol, LDL-cholesterol, and HDL-cholesterol, show some variation between groups. The high arsenic group generally has lower levels of total and LDL cholesterol, but HDL cholesterol levels are similar to those of the low arsenic group, though these differences do not reach statistical significance. Allostatic load scores are slightly lower in the high arsenic group compared to the low arsenic group. However, again, this difference is not statistically significant. This table provides a detailed overview of how elevated urinary arsenic levels correlate with specific clinical variables, highlighting that many of the differences, while present, do not achieve statistical significance.

Table 1. Clinical variables of interest in the study stratified by arsenic exposure levels

Variable Name	High Urinary Arsenic 50>mcg/L	Low Urinary Arsenic ≤50 mcg/L	p-value
Age in years at screening	52.08	43.57	0.001
Body Mass index	29.54	28.72	0.056
Average Systolic Blood Pressure	125.47	122.04	0.104
Average Diastolic Blood Pressure	71.29	71.56	0.311
Total cholesterol (mg/dL)	174.05	183.73	0.410
LDL-cholesterol (mg/dL)	99.38	107.99	0.307
HDL-cholesterol (mg/dL)	55.57	55.35	0.827
Allostatic Load	3.19	3.60	0.881
Triglyceride (mg/dL)	120.83	71.96	0.101

Figure 1 displays a Spearman Correlation Matrix, using a color gradient from green to red to illustrate the strength and direction of associations between a set of health-related variables. Green shades indicate positive correlations, while red shades represent negative correlations. The intensity of the color corresponds to the magnitude of the correlation, with darker shades indicating stronger correlations, whether positive or negative.

The matrix's diagonal, represented by the darkest green color, naturally shows a correlation of 1, as this is where each variable is paired with itself. Noteworthy within the matrix is the relationship between systolic blood pressure (SBP) and age, indicated by a lighter green color with a value of 0.5670, suggesting a moderately positive correlation rather than a negative one, meaning that higher SBP is associated with older age in this population.

The body mass index (BMI) has a moderate positive correlation with triglycerides, as evidenced by the value of 0.3532 and its corresponding green shade. This indicates that higher BMI is related to higher triglyceride levels in the individuals studied. In contrast, high-density lipoprotein cholesterol (HDL), commonly known as 'good cholesterol,' demonstrates a moderate negative correlation with triglycerides, marked by a value of -0.4736 and a reddish hue, suggesting that higher HDL levels are associated with lower triglyceride levels.

The matrix also shows that low-density lipoprotein cholesterol (LDL) is strongly positively correlated with total cholesterol, highlighted by a value of 0.9180 and a very dark green, denoting that LDL cholesterol levels are closely linked to total cholesterol levels in the subjects.

The arsenic variable shows relatively weak correlations with the other clinical variables, as evidenced by the pale colors in its row, with no strong positive or negative relationships standing out.

This matrix provides a visual and quantitative representation of the relationships between clinical variables, allowing for an immediate grasp of the potential interdependencies within this set of health-related data.

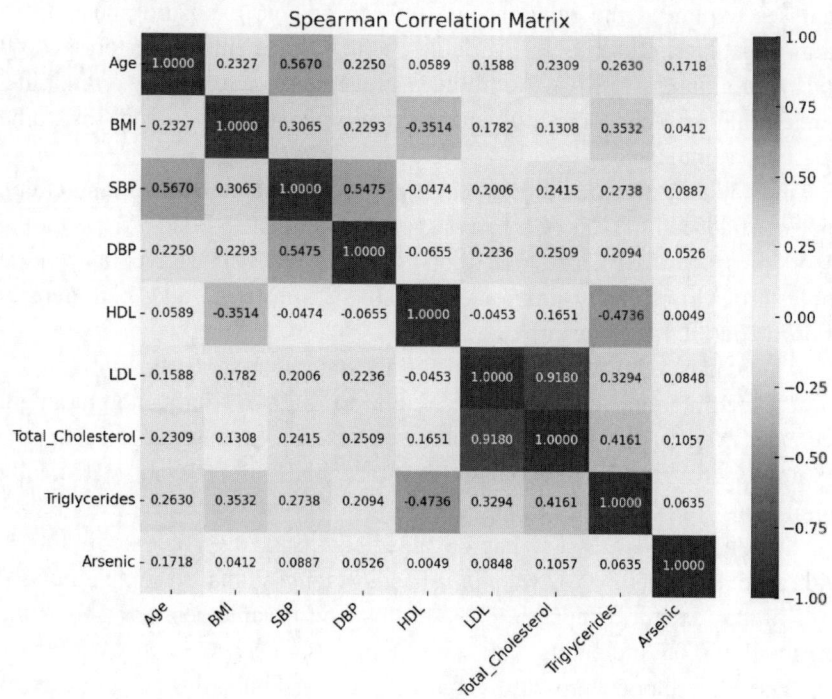

Figure 1. Correlation plot between predictor variables of interest.

Table 2. Simple linear regression of relationship between arsenic exposure and CVD variables. Association between total arsenic and variables of interest

Variables	*Arsenic Adjusted (95%CI)	p-Value
AL	-0.002(-0.005, -0.0001)	>0.05+
SBP	-0.013(-0.023, -0.001)	>0.05+
DBP	-0.005(0.016, 0.005)	>0.05
Triglycerides	0.049(-0.131, 0.229)	>0.05
Total Cholesterol	-0.010(-0.055, 0.034)	>0.05
LDL Cholesterol	-0.026(-0.117, 0.065)	>0.05
HDL Cholesterol	-0.005(-0.016, 0.005)	>0.05

*Adjusted for Age.
+Upon further adjustment for Urinary Creatinine, gender, BMI, Alcohol and Ethnicity.

Table 2 in the study provides results from simple linear regression analyses exploring the relationship between arsenic exposure and various cardiovascular disease (CVD) variables, with adjustments made for age and body mass index (BMI). Additional adjustments for urinary creatinine, gender, alcohol consumption, and Ethnicity have been made for some variables as indicated.

The table details the adjusted coefficients for arsenic with corresponding 95% confidence intervals (CIs) and p-values for allostatic load (AL), systolic blood pressure (SBP), diastolic blood pressure (DBP), triglycerides, total cholesterol, low-density lipoprotein (LDL) cholesterol, and high-density lipoprotein (HDL) cholesterol.

The arsenic adjusted coefficient for allostatic load is -0.002, with a 95% confidence interval ranging from -0.005 to -0.0001, indicating a slight decrease in allostatic load with increased arsenic exposure. However, the p-value is greater than 0.05, suggesting that this finding is not statistically significant.

Systolic blood pressure has an arsenic-adjusted coefficient of -0.013, with a 95% CI from -0.023 to -0.001, suggesting a small decrease in SBP with higher arsenic exposure. Despite this, the p-value remains above the threshold of 0.05, indicating a lack of statistical significance.

Diastolic blood pressure presents an arsenic-adjusted coefficient of -0.005, but the 95% CI crosses zero, from 0.016 to 0.005, which usually suggests a lack of a clear association. Consistent with this, the p-value is greater than 0.05, indicating no statistically significant relationship.

Triglycerides have an adjusted coefficient of 0.049 with a wide 95% CI from -0.131 to 0.229, and the p-value again is greater than 0.05, signifying no statistically significant association with arsenic exposure.

Total cholesterol, with an arsenic adjusted coefficient of -0.010 and a 95% CI from -0.055 to 0.034, along with LDL cholesterol, which has an adjusted coefficient of -0.026 and a 95% CI from -0.117 to 0.065, both show no significant relationship with arsenic exposure given their p-values greater than 0.05.

HDL cholesterol shows an adjusted coefficient of -0.005 with a 95% CI that includes zero, from -0.016 to 0.005, and like the other variables, the p-value exceeds 0.05, indicating that the relationship between HDL cholesterol levels and arsenic exposure is not statistically significant.

In summary, the analysis indicates that there is no statistically significant association within this dataset between arsenic exposure and the examined CVD variables when adjusted for the specified confounders.

Discussion

Our study aimed to explore the association between total urinary arsenic and various cardiovascular markers and allostatic load, hypothesizing that increased arsenic exposure might correlate with adverse cardiovascular outcomes and higher allostatic load, indicative of chronic stress. Contrary to our expectations and existing literature suggesting potential links between arsenic exposure and cardiovascular disease, our findings revealed no significant associations between total urinary arsenic levels and the cardiovascular markers or allostatic load.

The absence of a significant association between total arsenic and cardiovascular markers and allostatic load in our study could be attributed to several factors. Firstly, the use of total urinary arsenic as a biomarker for exposure may not precisely reflect the chronic exposure levels relevant to cardiovascular risk and allostatic load (31). Urinary arsenic predominantly captures recent exposure, and its levels can fluctuate significantly based on dietary intake, hydration status, and renal function (32). In contrast, blood arsenic might provide a more stable indicator of both acute and long-term exposure, potentially offering a clearer link to systemic effects and chronic conditions such as CVD (31).

Additionally, the specificity of arsenic species was not addressed in our study. Total urinary arsenic includes both inorganic arsenic, the more toxic form associated with health risks, and its metabolites and organic arsenic compounds commonly found in seafood, which are considered less harmful (33). The lack of speciation may have obscured the relationship between exposure to toxic arsenic species and cardiovascular health outcomes.

There was a signficant different between age and arsenic exposure with those having higher total arsenic exposure being significantly older. Arsenic, a ubiquitous environmental contaminant found in water, air, and soil, has well-documented toxic and carcinogenic effects, making its study crucial for understanding population risks.

The observed relationship between higher mean arsenic levels and older age could suggest several underlying dynamics. Older individuals may have had longer cumulative exposure durations, particularly in regions with historical arsenic contamination (34). This prolonged exposure could lead to higher body burdens of arsenic as evidenced by elevated mean levels in older populations. Additionally, changes in metabolic efficiency with age could alter the body's ability to detoxify and excrete arsenic, potentially leading to greater accumulation over time (35).

Furthermore, the patterns of arsenic exposure might also reflect changes in environmental regulations or shifts in industrial practices over the decades. Older generations might have been exposed to higher levels of arsenic during earlier years when environmental regulations were less stringent (36).

Our study speaks to the need for age-specific strategies in public health interventions and policy-making to mitigate arsenic exposure and its associated health risks. Historical and longitudinal exposure assessments are needed to address these issues fully.

Conclusion

Our findings, particularly the significant relationship between arsenic exposure and age, contribute to the broader discourse on environmental exposures and public health. They highlight the need for more nuanced research approaches, including arsenic speciation, long-term exposure assessment, and the consideration of individual susceptibility factors. Future studies should also investigate the potential cumulative effects of arsenic and other environmental agents on cardiovascular health and allostatic load across different life stages.

Acknowledgments

Conceptualization, E.O.-G.; methodology, E.O.-G; formal analysis, E.B., E.O.-G..; investigation, E.B., E.O.-G.; resources, E.O.-G.; data curation, E.O.-G.; writing—original draft preparation, E.B, and E.O.-G.; writing—review and editing, E.B., E.O.-G; supervision, E.O.-G.; project administration, E.O.-G.; funding acquisition, E.O.-G. All authors have read and agreed to the published version of the manuscript.

Funding

Research reported in this publication was supported by the National Institute of General Medical Sciences of the National Institutes of Health under Award Number R16GM149473. The content is solely the responsibility of the authors and does not necessarily represent the official views of the National Institutes of Health.

References

[1] Gaidai O, Cao Y, Loginov S. Global cardiovascular diseases death rate prediction. Curr Probl Cardiol 2023;48(5):101622.
[2] Forman DE, Rich MW, Alexander KP, Zieman S, Maurer MS, Najjar SS, et al. Cardiac care for older adults: time for a new paradigm. J Am Coll Cardiol 2011;57(18):1801-10.
[3] Flora GD, Nayak MK. A brief review of cardiovascular diseases, associated risk factors and current treatment regimes. Curr Pharm Des 2019;25(38):4063-84.
[4] van Wyk JT, van Wijk MA, Sturkenboom MC, Moorman PW, van der Lei J. Identification of the four conventional cardiovascular disease risk factors by Dutch general practitioners. Chest 2005;128(4):2521-7.
[5] Juarez PD, Hood DB, Song M-A, Ramesh A. Use of an exposome approach to understand the effects of exposures from the natural, built, and social environments on cardio-vascular disease onset, progression, and outcomes. Front Public Health 2020;8:379.
[6] Teshale AB, Htun HL, Owen A, Gasevic D, Phyo AZZ, Fancourt D, et al. The role of social determinants of health in cardiovascular diseases: An umbrella review. J Am Heart Assoc 2023;12(13):e029765.
[7] Obeng-Gyasi E. Lead exposure and oxidative stress—A life course approach in US adults. Toxics 2018;6(3):42.

[8] Obeng-Gyasi E, Roostaei J, Gibson JM. Lead distribution in urban soil in a medium-Sized City: Household-scale analysis. Environ Sci Technol 2021;55(6):3696-705.
[9] Vaziri ND. Mechanisms of lead-induced hypertension and cardiovascular disease. Am J Physiol Heart Circ Physiol 2008;295(2):H454-65.
[10] Cañas Portilla AI, Castaño A, Organization WH. Human health effects of benzene, arsenic, cadmium, nickel, lead and mercury: Report of an expert consultation. Geneva: World Health Organization, 2024.
[11] Rossman TG. Mechanism of arsenic carcinogenesis: an integrated approach. Mutat Res 2003;533(1-2):37-65.
[12] Benbrahim-Tallaa L, Waalkes MP. Inorganic arsenic and human prostate cancer. Environ Health Perspect 2008;116(2):158-64.
[13] Kwok RK, Kaufmann RB, Jakariya M. Arsenic in drinking-water and reproductive health outcomes: A study of participants in the Bangladesh Integrated Nutrition Programme. J Health Popult Nutr 2006;24(2):190-205.
[14] Sharma A, Kumar S. Arsenic exposure with reference to neurological impairment: An overview. Rev Environ Health 2019;34(4):403-14.
[15] Hong Y-S, Song K-H, Chung J-Y. Health effects of chronic arsenic exposure. J Prev Med Public Health 2014;47(5):245.
[16] States JC, Srivastava S, Chen Y, Barchowsky A. Arsenic and cardiovascular disease. Toxicol Sci 2009,107(2):312-23.
[17] Jomova K, Jenisova Z, Feszterova M, Baros S, Liska J, Hudecova D, et al. Arsenic: Toxicity, oxidative stress and human disease. J Appl Toxicol 2011;31(2):95-107.
[18] Rahman M, Sohel N, Yunus M, Chowdhury ME, Hore SK, Zaman K, et al. A prospective cohort study of stroke mortality and arsenic in drinking water in Bangladeshi adults. BMC Public Health 2014;14:1-8.
[19] Lantz RC, Hays AM. Role of oxidative stress in arsenic-induced toxicity. Drug Metab Rev 2006;38(4):791-804.
[20] Gump BB, Heffernan K, Brann LS, Hill DT, Labrie-Cleary C, Jandev V, et al. Exposure to arsenic and subclinical cardiovascular disease in 9-to 11-year-old children, Syracuse, New York. JAMA Network Open 2023;6(6):e2321379.
[21] McEwen BS. Stress, adaptation, and disease: Allostasis and allostatic load. Ann NY Acad Sci 1998;840(1):33-44.
[22] McEwen BS. Protection and damage from acute and chronic stress: allostasis and allostatic overload and relevance to the pathophysiology of psychiatric disorders. Ann NY Acad Sci 2004;1032(1):1-7.
[23] McEwen BS, Gianaros PJ. Central role of the brain in stress and adaptation: links to socioeconomic status, health, and disease. Ann NY Acad Sci 2010;1186(1):190-222.
[24] Obeng-Gyasi E, Ferguson AC, Stamatakis KA, Province MA. Combined effect of lead exposure and allostatic load on cardiovascular disease mortality—A preliminary study. Int J Environ Res Public Health 2021;18(13):6879.
[25] Logan JG, Barksdale DJ. Allostasis and allostatic load: expanding the discourse on stress and cardiovascular disease. J Clin Nurs 2008;17(7b):201-8.

[26] Centers for Disease Control and Prevention. Laboratory procedure manual. URL: https://wwwn.cdc.gov/nchs/data/nhanes/2015-2016/labmethods/PFAS_I_MET.pdf.
[27] McEwen BS. Mood disorders and allostatic load. Biol Psychiatry 2003;54(3):200-7.
[28] Obeng-Gyasi E, Obeng-Gyasi B. Chronic stress and cardiovascular disease among individuals exposed to lead: A pilot study. Diseases 2020;8(1):7.
[29] Hill M, Obeng-Gyasi E. The association of cytomegalovirus IgM and allostatic load. Diseases 2022;10(4):70.
[30] Boafo YS, Mostafa S, Obeng-Gyasi E. Association of combined metals and PFAS with cardiovascular disease risk. Toxics 2023;11(12):979.
[31] Hall M, Chen Y, Ahsan H, Slavkovich V, Van Geen A, Parvez F, et al. Blood arsenic as a biomarker of arsenic exposure: results from a prospective study. Toxicology 2006;225(2-3):225-33.
[32] Marchiset-Ferlay N, Savanovitch C, Sauvant-Rochat M-P. What is the best biomarker to assess arsenic exposure via drinking water? Environ Int 2012;39(1):150-71.
[33] Hughes MF. Biomarkers of exposure: A case study with inorganic arsenic. Environ Health Perspect 2006;114(11):1790-6.
[34] Ferrario D, Gribaldo L, Hartung T. Arsenic exposure and immunotoxicity: a review including the possible influence of age and sex. Curr Environ Health Rep 2016;3:1-12.
[35] Lindberg A-L, Ekström E-C, Nermell B, Rahman M, Lönnerdal B, Persson L-Å, et al. Gender and age differences in the metabolism of inorganic arsenic in a highly exposed population in Bangladesh. Environ Res 2008;106(1):110-20.
[36] Parascandola J. King of poisons: A history of arsenic. Lincoln, NE: Potomac Books, 2012.

Section Two: Acknowledgments

Chapter 8

About the Authors

Emmanuel Obeng-Gyasi, PhD, MPH, is Associate Professor at the Department of Built Environment and [2]Environmental Health and Disease Laboratory, North Carolina A&T State University, Greensboro, North Carolina, United States of America. His research interests encompass investigating the effects of environmental agents on both the environment and populations using biostatistics/epidemiology, molecular biology and analytical chemistry techniques. His primary focus is on the exposome, which represents the sum of all environmental exposures across an individual's life course. Within this domain, he specializes in studying the health effects of multi-pollutant mixtures, metals, per- and polyfluoroalkyl substances (PFAS), and persistent infections. In his lab, he is dedicated to developing and applying analytic approaches for assessing chemical mixtures. His research also extends to examining the intersection of environmental exposures with social factors. This exploration aims to achieve a better understanding of the complex interplay between stress arousal and environmental agents, ultimately shedding light on potential disparities in health outcomes among different social groups. Email: eobenggyasi@ncat.edu

Joav Merrick, MD, MMedSci, DMSc, born and educated in Denmark, is Professor of Pediatrics, Division of Pediatrics, Hadassah Hebrew University Medical Center, Mt Scopus Campus, Jerusalem, Israel and Kentucky Children's Hospital, University of Kentucky, Lexington, Kentucky United States and professor of public health at the Center for Healthy Development, School of Public Health, Georgia State University, Atlanta, United States, the former medical director of the Health Services, Division for Intellectual

In: Public Health: Understanding the Impact of Environmental Pollutants
Editors: Emmanuel Obeng-Gyasi and Joav Merrick
ISBN: 979-8-89530-579-9
© 2025 Nova Science Publishers, Inc.

and Developmental Disabilities, Ministry of Social Affairs and Social Services, Jerusalem, the founder and director of the National Institute of Child Health and Human Development in Israel. Numerous publications in the field of pediatrics, child health and human development, rehabilitation, intellectual disability, disability, health, welfare, abuse, advocacy, quality of life and prevention. Received the Peter Sabroe Child Award for outstanding work on behalf of Danish Children in 1985 and the International LEGO-Prize ("The Children's Nobel Prize") for an extraordinary contribution towards improvement in child welfare and well-being in 1987. In 2017 appointed a Kentucky Colonel by the Commonwealth of Kentucky, the highest honor the governor can bestow to a person.
Email: jmerrick@zahav.net.il

Chapter 9

About the Department of Built Environment, North Carolina A&T State University, Greensboro and Environmental Health and Disease Laboratory, North Carolina A&T State University, Greensboro, North Carolina, United States of America

The Department of Built Environment at North Carolina A&T State University, housed within the College of Science and Technology, offers specialized programs in Construction Management, Environmental Health and Safety, and Geomatics. These programs provide a comprehensive education, integrating academic rigor with hands-on industry experience. The department also collaborates on a shared Master's degree and contributes to the Applied Science and Technology Ph.D. program. Environmental Health and Safety offers an undergraduate certificate, and both Environmental Health and Geomatics programs provide online degree options. Research within the department focuses on sustainable construction, occupational health, geospatial sciences, and environmental risk assessment.

The Environmental Health and Disease Laboratory plays a crucial role in studying environmental exposures and their impact on public health, fostering interdisciplinary collaboration. It is a community-engaged field research and data analytics laboratory dedicated to investigating exposures at the household, neighborhood, and broader scales. The lab employs advanced methodologies to analyze environmental contaminants, assess distribution patterns, and explore their effects on human health. By integrating field studies, laboratory analysis, and statistical modeling, lab researchers aim to provide data-driven insights that inform public health policies and

In: Public Health: Understanding the Impact of Environmental Pollutants
Editors: Emmanuel Obeng-Gyasi and Joav Merrick
ISBN: 979-8-89530-579-9
© 2025 Nova Science Publishers, Inc.

interventions. Through partnerships with local communities, governmental agencies, and academic institutions, the lab actively contributes to addressing environmental health challenges and promoting healthier living conditions.

Chapter 10

About the National Institute of Child Health and Human Development in Israel

The National Institute of Child Health and Human Development (NICHD) in Israel was established in 1998 as a virtual institute under the auspicies of the Medical Director, Ministry of Social Affairs and Social Services in order to function as the research arm for the Office of the Medical Director. In 1998 the National Council for Child Health and Pediatrics, Ministry of Health and in 1999 the Director General and Deputy Director General of the Ministry of Health endorsed the establishment of the NICHD.

Mission

The mission of a National Institute for Child Health and Human Development in Israel is to provide an academic focal point for the scholarly interdisciplinary study of child life, health, public health, welfare, disability, rehabilitation, intellectual disability and related aspects of human development. This mission includes research, teaching, clinical work, information and public service activities in the field of child health and human development.

Service and academic activities

Over the years many activities became focused in the south of Israel due to collaboration with various professionals at the Faculty of Health Sciences (FOHS) at the Ben Gurion University of the Negev (BGU). Since 2000 an affiliation with the Zusman Child Development Center at the Pediatric

In: Public Health: Understanding the Impact of Environmental Pollutants
Editors: Emmanuel Obeng-Gyasi and Joav Merrick
ISBN: 979-8-89530-579-9
© 2025 Nova Science Publishers, Inc.

Division of Soroka University Medical Center has resulted in collaboration around the establishment of the Down Syndrome Clinic at that center. In 2002 a full course on "Disability" was established at the Recanati School for Allied Professions in the Community, FOHS, BGU and in 2005 collaboration was started with the Primary Care Unit of the faculty and disability became part of the master of public health course on "Children and society". In the academic year 2005-2006 a one semester course on "Aging with disability" was started as part of the master of science program in gerontology in our collaboration with the Center for Multidisciplinary Research in Aging. In 2010 collaborations with the Division of Pediatrics, Hadassah Hebrew University Medical Center, Jerusalem, Israel around the National Down Syndrome Center and teaching students and residents about intellectual and developmental disabilities as part of their training at this campus.

Research activities

The affiliated staff have over the years published work from projects and research activities in this national and international collaboration. In the year 2000 the International Journal of Adolescent Medicine and Health and in 2005 the International Journal on Disability and Human Development of De Gruyter Publishing House (Berlin and New York) were affiliated with the National Institute of Child Health and Human Development. From 2008 also the International Journal of Child Health and Human Development (Nova Science, New York), the International Journal of Child and Adolescent Health (Nova Science) and the Journal of Pain Management (Nova Science) affiliated and from 2009 the International Public Health Journal (Nova Science) and Journal of Alternative Medicine Research (Nova Science). All peer-reviewed international journals.

National collaborations

Nationally the NICHD works in collaboration with the Faculty of Health Sciences, Ben Gurion University of the Negev; Department of Physical Therapy, Sackler School of Medicine, Tel Aviv University; Autism Center, Assaf HaRofeh Medical Center; National Rett and PKU Centers at Chaim

Sheba Medical Center, Tel HaShomer; Department of Physiotherapy, Haifa University; Department of Education, Bar Ilan University, Ramat Gan, Faculty of Social Sciences and Health Sciences; College of Judea and Samaria in Ariel and in 2011 affiliation with Center for Pediatric Chronic Diseases and National Center for Down Syndrome, Department of Pediatrics, Hadassah Hebrew University Medical Center, Mount Scopus Campus, Jerusalem.

International collaborations

Internationally with the Department of Disability and Human Development, College of Applied Health Sciences, University of Illinois at Chicago; Strong Center for Developmental Disabilities, Golisano Children's Hospital at Strong, University of Rochester School of Medicine and Dentistry, New York; Centre on Intellectual Disabilities, University of Albany, New York; Centre for Chronic Disease Prevention and Control, Health Canada, Ottawa; Chandler Medical Center and Children's Hospital, Kentucky Children's Hospital, Section of Adolescent Medicine, University of Kentucky, Lexington; Chronic Disease Prevention and Control Research Center, Baylor College of Medicine, Houston, Texas; Division of Neuroscience, Department of Psychiatry, Columbia University, New York; Institute for the Study of Disadvantage and Disability, Atlanta; Center for Autism and Related Disorders, Department Psychiatry, Children's Hospital Boston, Boston; Department of Pediatric and Adolescent Medicine, Western Michigan University Homer Stryker MD School of Medicine, Kalamazoo, Michigan, United States; Department of Paediatrics, Child Health and Adolescent Medicine, Children's Hospital at Westmead, Westmead, Australia; International Centre for the Study of Occupational and Mental Health, Düsseldorf, Germany; Centre for Advanced Studies in Nursing, Department of General Practice and Primary Care, University of Aberdeen, Aberdeen, United Kingdom; Quality of Life Research Center, Copenhagen, Denmark; Nordic School of Public Health, Gottenburg, Sweden, Scandinavian Institute of Quality of Working Life, Oslo, Norway; The Department of Applied Social Sciences (APSS) of The Hong Kong Polytechnic University Hong Kong.

Targets

Our focus is on research, international collaborations, clinical work, teaching and policy in health, disability and human development and to establish the NICHD as a permanent institute in Israel in order to conduct model research and policy.

Contact

Professor Joav Merrick, MD, MMedSci, DMSc
Director, National Institute of Child Health and Human Development, Jerusalem, Israel.
E-mail: jmerrick@zahav.net.il

Section Three: Index

Index

A

accuracy, 32, 33, 34, 37, 39, 41, 51
air quality, 5, 6, 9, 12, 20, 22, 23, 24, 32, 35, 44, 47, 48, 86, 89, 103
air quality monitoring, 22, 47, 48
air quality monitors, 6, 9, 44
albumin, 115, 116, 119, 120, 129, 137, 138
allostatic load (AL), 12, 33, 35, 46, 47, 48, 49, 50, 51, 52, 53, 74, 80, 81, 82, 83, 86, 87, 93, 94, 95, 96, 97, 98, 110, 111, 113, 115, 116, 117, 118, 119, 120, 121, 122, 123, 124, 125, 126, 127, 128, 129, 130, 131, 134, 135, 136, 137, 138, 139, 140, 142, 143, 144,145, 146, 147
amperometric sensors, 26
arsenic, iv, 3, 4, 31, 38, 50, 114, 127, 131, 133, 134, 135, 136, 137, 139, 140, 141, 142, 143, 144, 146, 147
arsenic exposure 131, 133, 134, 135, 136, 137, 140, 142, 143, 144, 146, 147
atmospheric pollutants, 23, 24

B

biological hazards, 58, 59, 69, 70, 71, 81, 82
biomarkers, 4, 97, 120, 128, 130, 131, 138, 147
body mass index (BMI), 115, 116, 119, 120, 121, 123, 128, 137, 138, 139, 140, 142
built environment, 3, 9, 38, 47, 52, 55, 78, 85, 99, 113, 131, 151, 153

C

cadmium, 51, 87, 88, 89, 91, 96, 114, 127, 133, 146
calcium, 38, 102, 108
cancers, 56, 73, 86, 87, 95, 133
carbon monoxide (CO), 14, 15, 23, 38, 70, 85, 86, 88, 91, 100, 118, 132, 137
cardiovascular disease (CVD), 4, 5, 19, 37, 38, 39, 52, 56, 73, 80, 81, 96, 113, 114, 115, 117, 120, 123, 124, 126, 127, 128, 129, 130, 131, 132, 133, 134, 135, 136, 142, 143, 145, 146, 147
cardiovascular disease risk, 96, 113, 117, 120, 124, 126, 127, 129, 131, 134, 136, 145, 147
cardiovascular health, 36, 37, 52, 113, 124, 125, 126, 134, 136, 144
cardiovascular health monitoring, 36
cardiovascular risks, 4
central nervous system, 102, 106, 114
chemical hazards, 55, 58, 59, 65, 72, 73, 74, 82
chemiresistive sensing, 28
chemiresistive-based sensors, 28
chronic obstructive pulmonary disease (COPD), 80, 85, 87, 89, 90, 91, 92, 93, 96
Clean Air Act, 103, 108, 111
cognitive ability, 102
community partnerships, 44
contaminants, 19, 24, 26, 31, 49, 85, 91, 92
continuous glucose monitoring (CGM), 35, 50

C-reactive protein (CRP), 96, 115, 116, 117, 118, 119, 120, 121, 122, 123, 124, 126, 128, 136, 137, 138
creatinine clearance, 115, 116, 119, 120, 137, 138
cyber security threats, 39

D

data privacy, 10, 39, 43, 45
diabetes, 34, 35, 36, 37, 50, 51, 114, 128, 129, 132, 134
diastolic blood pressure (DBP), 113, 115, 116, 117, 118, 119, 121, 122, 123, 124, 126, 136, 137, 138, 142
digital divide, 40, 53
digital literacy, 43, 53
digital systems, 43
disability status, 15
discrimination, 16, 18, 19, 20, 30, 61

E

electrochemical sensors, 26, 28
employment, 18, 19, 21, 43, 62, 65, 76, 77, 82
environmental contaminants, 3, 4, 87, 88, 91, 92, 93, 135, 153
environmental data, 9, 41
environmental disparity, 15
environmental justice (EJ), 5, 9, 10, 11, 14, 15, 20, 21, 34, 44, 45, 46, 50, 51, 52, 96
environmental monitoring, 5, 11, 12, 22, 29, 32, 39, 41, 47, 49, 50
environmental pollutants, 3, 4, 5, 11, 34, 35, 86
environmental pollution, 12, 21, 38, 93, 108
ethical considerations, 41
ethical data collection, 43
ethnicity, 15, 139, 142

G

geographical location, 15

H

health equity, 5, 77
health implications, 11, 58, 100, 102, 108, 116, 131
health monitoring, 14, 34, 45
health outcomes, 3, 4, 6, 16, 24, 57, 65, 77, 79, 86, 95, 126, 134, 146, 151
health tracking, 34
heart rate (HR), 13, 14, 36, 40, 51, 52
heavy metals, 27, 38, 73, 85, 87, 88, 89, 91, 92, 97, 114, 127
hemoglobin A1C, 119, 128, 137, 138
high-density lipoprotein (HDL) cholesterol, 115, 116, 118, 119, 120, 121, 122, 123, 124, 129, 136, 137, 138, 139, 140, 142, 143

I

industrial zones, 21, 133

J

Jackson, Mississippi, 99, 100, 101, 109, 110

L

land use policies, 18
laptops, 23
lead (Pb), 4, 5, 18, 19, 20, 23, 34, 36, 38, 39, 51, 65, 68, 70, 73, 87, 88, 89, 91, 92, 96, 97, 98, 99, 100, 101, 102, 103, 104, 105, 106, 107, 108, 109, 110, 111, 114, 116, 117, 127, 129, 133, 137, 144, 145, 146, 147
lead (Pb) contamination, 100, 101, 103, 106, 107, 108, 110
lead control, 103
lead poisoning, 102, 105, 110, 111
lead pollution, 99, 100, 101, 110
low-density lipoprotein (LDL) cholesterol, 113, 115, 117, 118, 121, 122, 123, 124, 126, 129, 136, 137, 139, 140, 141, 142, 143

Index

M

marginalized communities, 9, 11, 12, 13, 15, 17, 21, 22, 24, 28, 30, 36, 40, 41, 42, 45, 108
mercury, 3, 4, 36, 87, 88, 89, 91, 96, 113, 114, 115, 116, 117, 118, 119, 120, 121, 122, 123, 124, 125, 126, 127, 128, 129, 130, 133, 146
mercury exposure, 4, 96, 113, 115, 116, 117, 118, 120, 123, 124, 125, 126, 127, 128, 129, 130
mercury levels, 113, 115, 116, 117, 118, 120, 122, 123, 124
metals, 36, 38, 51, 85, 87, 88, 89, 90, 91, 92, 96, 97, 102, 108, 114, 129, 133, 147, 151
micro-chips, 12
mobile crowdsensing (MCS), 32, 50

N

nitrogen, 23, 38
noise mapping, 31, 33, 50
noise pollution monitors, 31

O

obesity, 37, 38, 52, 127, 128
occupational environments, 4, 71
occupational exposures, 3, 4, 5, 57, 78, 86, 95
occupational hazards, 55, 56, 58, 59, 60, 61, 72, 76, 77, 78, 79
occupational health outcomes, 76
occupational health promotion, 56, 59, 77
occupational health protection, 56, 77
occupational health risks, 4, 58
organizational factors, 61, 76, 83
ozone, 23, 38

P

particulate matter, 23, 24, 38, 46, 86, 93, 94
PFAS (per- and polyfluoroalkyl substances), 75, 83, 85, 86, 87, 88, 90, 91, 92, 94, 95, 96, 97, 129, 147, 151
physical hazards, 58, 59, 65, 81
political influence, 20
polychlorinated biphenyls (PCBs), 10, 11, 35, 46, 103
polycyclic aromatic hydrocarbons, 86
potentiometric sensors, 26, 27
psychosocial stresses, 5
public health, 3, 4, 5, 6, 9, 24, 25, 44, 45, 50, 51, 57, 63, 67, 79, 80, 81, 83, 85, 88, 89, 92, 94, 95, 96, 98, 99, 100, 101, 103, 105, 108, 109, 110, 111, 127, 128, 129, 130, 135, 136, 144, 145, 146, 151, 153, 155, 156, 157
public health monitoring, 9, 44

R

respiratory health, 85, 86, 87, 88, 89, 91, 92, 93, 94, 95

S

safe drinking water, 30, 100, 101, 103, 108, 110, 111
Safe Drinking Water Act, 101, 103, 108, 110, 111
security, 10, 39, 43, 45, 53, 65, 76, 78
single-wall carbon nanotubes (SWCNTs), 28, 49
skin cancer, 19, 25, 34, 48
smart clothes, 14
smart earphones, 14
smart glasses, 13, 14
smart shoes, 14
smart tattoos, 12
smartphones, 13, 23, 32, 42
smartwatches, 13
social determinants of health (SDOH), 65, 78, 79, 80, 83, 108, 145
socioeconomic factors, 55, 59, 76, 77
socioeconomic status, 11, 15, 47, 58, 65, 77, 78, 83, 108, 128, 130, 146
sulfur dioxide (SO_2), 23, 38

systemic disparity, 15
systemic racism, 16, 17, 18, 19, 21, 47
systolic blood pressure (SBP), 117, 118, 119, 121, 122, 123, 124, 136, 137, 140, 142

T

technological accessibility, 39, 40, 45
total cholesterol, 113, 115, 116, 117, 118, 119, 120, 121, 122, 123, 124, 126, 136, 137, 138, 139, 140, 141, 142, 143
toxic chemicals, 5, 10, 56, 60, 73
Toxic Substances Control Act, 103, 108, 111
triglycerides, 113, 115, 116, 117, 118, 119, 120, 122, 123, 124, 126, 128, 136, 137, 138, 140, 142, 143

U

ultraviolet (UV) exposure sensors, 9, 25, 44
United States Environmental Protection Agency (EPA), 10, 31, 100, 101, 103, 108, 109, 110, 111, 115
urbanization, 32, 100
UV exposure sensors, 9, 44

V

validity, 41, 53
vitamin D, 25
volatile organic compounds (VOCs), 23, 86, 94

W

waste management, 15, 70, 116, 133
water quality, 9, 12, 26, 27, 28, 29, 30, 44, 48, 49
water quality monitoring (WQM), 27, 28, 29, 48, 49
water quality sensors, 9, 26, 44
water shortage, 99
wealth gap, 19
wearable devices, 5, 6, 9, 12, 13, 14, 15, 22, 23, 34, 36, 39, 40, 41, 43, 44, 45, 46, 47, 51, 52, 53
wearable sensor technologies, 9
wearable technologies, 9, 12, 53
wearable UV sensors, 25
wearables, 12, 13, 40, 41, 43, 44, 45, 53
worker health, 4

Z

zoning, 18, 19, 21